Susan Gardiner, MD
Albany Medical Center
ID & DEA Number: 61706

MANUAL OF
ADMITTING
ORDERS
AND
THERAPEUTICS

MANUAL OF

ADMITTING

ORDERS

AND

THERAPEUTICS

Third Edition

ERIC B. LARSON, M.D., M.P.H.

Professor, Department of Medicine
University of Washington;
Medical Director
University of Washington Medical Center
Seattle, Washington

W. CONRAD LILES, Jr., M.D., Ph.D.

Senior Fellow in Allergy and Infectious Diseases
Acting Instructor in Medicine
Department of Medicine
University of Washington
Seattle, Washington

W.B. SAUNDERS COMPANY
A Division of Harcourt Brace & Company

PHILADELPHIA · LONDON · TORONTO · MONTREAL · SYDNEY · TOKYO

W.B. SAUNDERS COMPANY
A Division of
Harcourt Brace & Company

The Curtis Center
Independence Square West
Philadelphia, Pennsylvania 19106

Library of Congress Cataloging-in-Publication Data

Larson, Eric B.

Manual of admitting orders and therapeutics / Eric B. Larson, W. Conrad
Liles, Jr.—3rd ed.

   p.   cm.

Includes index.

ISBN 0-7216-5268-9

1. Hospital care—Handbooks, manuals, etc.   2. Hospitals—Admission
and discharge—Handbooks, manuals, etc.   3. Therapeutics—
Handbooks, manuals, etc.   I. Liles, W. Conrad, Jr.   II. Title.

[DNLM: 1. Patient Admission—handbooks.   2. Therapeutics—
handbooks.   3. Admitting Department, Hospital—organization &
administration—handbooks.   4. Hospital Administration—handbooks.
WX 39 L334m 1994]

RA972.L28   1994

362.1'1'0685—dc20

DNLM/DLC   93–26134

Manual of Admitting Orders and Therapeutics   ISBN 0–7216–5268–9

Printed in the United States of America

Last digit is the print number: 9   8   7   6   5   4   3   2

PREFACE

INTRODUCTION

The writing of medical orders is a skill that is usually taught to third- and fourth-year medical students by junior house staff. During the first days of a medicine or surgery clerkship, the intern or resident typically sits down with the student to demonstrate how he or she writes orders; the student is expected to do them similarly. The end result depends on a variety of circumstances, including the skills and patience of the house officer, the demands of clinical work, the time available for teaching, and the work habits of the student.

It was no doubt such haphazard and inconsistent instruction that prompted a former medical student, Dr. Nicholas Juele, to suggest this manual. He expressed dismay and regret that there was no text on the writing of admitting orders. He felt that a manual could be used by students, house staff, practicing physicians, nursing staff, and pharmacists to foster more effective communication in the medical order book.

Once we ourselves became aware of this need, we were astounded by the number of physicians, house staff, nurses, ward clerks, and pharmacists with similar concerns. Furthermore, a 1979 review of the medical order writing practices in our hospitals revealed the lack of a systematic approach, with orders frequently being written ambiguously and a general lack of concern for this important means of communication.

Orders for intravenous fluids were singled out for special study in a university hospital audit. The result revealed that substantial numbers of orders were ambiguously or improperly written. Substantial losses occurred because intravenous fluids were returned unused daily to the pharmacy because of improperly written orders. The study concluded that ambiguous orders led to unnecessary waste, extra work for staff, and confusion in patient care.

PURPOSE

This manual presents an approach and a guide to medical order writing. The approach is best illustrated by sample admitting orders for commonly encountered medical illnesses. The illnesses used as examples were selected from a list of the most common discharge diagnoses encountered in the medical service of the teaching hospitals of the University of Washington. For the third edition, "new" diagnoses have been added to reflect changing patterns of illness in the community. The orders are accompanied by a narrative that is designed to explain the rationale behind each order. We hope that the narrative will also provide the reader with insights into patient care and the specific illnesses being discussed. A section on therapeutic agents also has been written and can serve as a convenient, up-to-date source of information for those writing medication orders.

We have chosen to approach medical order writing using admitting orders as models. Admitting orders are necessary for every hospitalized patient and are usually the most complete and detailed orders that are written. These will undoubtedly be revised and updated frequently, especially for seriously ill patients. In addition, orders are not necessarily written, but may be given verbally, to be transcribed and signed later. The principles illustrated by the admitting orders contained in this book provide an approach that is applicable to all aspects of medical order writing, including revisions and updates of original orders and verbal orders.

The *Manual of Admitting Orders and Therapeutics* is not a textbook of medicine nor is it a manual of medical therapeutics. Although we hope that the reader will learn something about medical diseases and their treatment from this book, one will not find sufficient information to use this book in lieu of a comprehensive textbook of medicine.

ORGANIZATION

Part I offers an approach to writing admitting orders and a discussion of the components of "perfect" admitting orders. Part II presents examples of admitting orders for over 70 common medical conditions. Part III contains orders that might be written for commonly performed procedures. Part IV provides prescribing information for over 500 drugs.

The absence of surgical orders does not indicate that surgical orders are less important or any easier to write clearly. The exclusion merely reflects our training, experience, and current practice. The principles illustrated apply equally to orders for surgical patients.

Finally, drug dosages, indications, and side effects are based on the most up-to-date information available to us at the time of printing. Drug dosages and indications change as a result of laboratory and clinical studies, and additional side effects are appreciated with further experience. For this reason, we encourage the reader to check package insert information for the manufacturers' recommended dosages.

THIRD EDITION

The third edition has been completely updated to reflect the changing practice of medicine. Specific admitting orders have been expanded to include three new sections on AIDS, new sections on unstable angina and on spinal cord compression. Detailed changes have been made within the existing chapters to reflect the most recent standard of care and changes in our understanding of the rationale for various medical orders. Drugs and procedures that are no longer used have been deleted. The section on drugs (Section IV) has been completely revised to reflect major advances in pharmacotherapeutics since publication of the second edition in 1987. The changes were made as a result of changes that have occurred in medical practice and, equally important, as a result of requests for new material from residents, practitioners, students, and pharmacists who have used the first two editions.

ACKNOWLEDGMENTS

We especially acknowledge the significant contributions of Mickey Eisenberg, M.D., as coauthor of the first two editions. We continue to be grateful to Jack Hanley, who served as the original catalyst for the manual, and to John Dyson, now retired senior editor at W.B. Saunders Company, who has been a long-standing supporter and source of encouragement for this manual. We also thank colleagues who have contributed and provided advice and assistance in earlier additions, including Tim Chestnut, Sue Heckbert, John Olsen, Gerald Bernstein, and Gerald Segal.

ERIC B. LARSON

W. CONRAD LILES, JR.

CONTENTS

LIST OF ABBREVIATIONS

ABGs	arterial blood gases
a.c.	ante cibum (before meals)
ACTH	adrenocorticotropic hormone
ADH	antidiuretic hormone
ad lib	ad libitum (at pleasure, freely)
AFB	acid-fast bacillus
alk phos	alkaline phosphatase
ALT	alanine aminotransferase
amp	ampule
AMV	assisted mandatory ventilation; assist mode ventilation
ANA	antinuclear antibody
anti-HAA	antibody hepatitis-associated antigen
AP	anteroposterior
ARDS	adult respiratory distress syndrome
ASA	acetylsalicylic acid
AST	aspartate aminotransferase
B-12	vitamin B-12 (cyanocobalamin)
b.i.d.	bis in die (twice a day)
BM	bowel movement
BP	blood pressure
BUN	blood urea nitrogen
$\bar{c}$	cum (with)
C	centigrade
C and S	culture and sensitivity
C3, C4	third and fourth complement components
Ca, Ca^{++}	calcium
cap	capsule
CBC	complete blood count, including hemoglobin, hematocrit, red cell indices, white blood cell count, and platelet estimation
CCU	coronary care unit
CH_{50}	total serum hemolytic complements
CMF	cyclophosphamide, methotrexate, and fluorouracil
CNS	central nervous system
CO_2	carbon dioxide
COPD	chronic obstructive pulmonary disease
CPK	creatinine phosphokinase

CPK-MB	creatine phosphokinase-myocardial band or myocardial-specific CPK isoenzyme (also CPK-2)
CPR	cardiopulmonary resuscitation
CSF	cerebrospinal fluid
CT	computerized tomography
CVA	cerebrovascular accident
CVP	central venous pressure
CXR	chest x-ray
D5	5% dextrose solution; also D10, D50, and so on
d/c	discharge; discontinue
DIC	disseminated intravascular coagulation
diff	differential count
DKA	diabetic ketoacidosis
dl	deciliter
DNA	deoxyribonucleic acid
DOSS	docusate sodium sulfosuccinate—a stool softener
DTs	delirium tremens
ECG	electrocardiogram
electrolytes	serum sodium, potassium, chloride bicarbonate concentration
ER	emergency room
ERCP	endoscopic retrograde cholangiopancreatography
ESR	erythrocyte sedimentation rate
ET	endotracheal tube
Fe/TIBC	iron/total iron-binding capacity
FEV_1	forced expiratory volume (in one second)
FiO_2	fractional inspired oxygen
5-FU	fluorouracil
g	gram(s)
GC	gonococcal; gonococcus
GFR	glomerular filtration rate
GI	gastrointestinal
glu	glucose
h	hour(s)
HB_sAG	hepatitis B surface antigen
HCO_3	bicarbonate
Hct	hematocrit
HDL	high-density lipoprotein
Hg	mercury
Hgb	hemoglobin concentration
hs	hora somni (hour of sleep, at bedtime)
HP	high potency
HTLV	human T cell lymphotropic virus
I and O	intake and output—measurement of the patient's intake by any route (mouth, vein, rectum) and output by any route, including urine, vomit, diarrhea, and fluid removed or lost from bleeding or body cavities
ICU	intensive care unit

IgM	immunoglobulin M
IMV	intermittent mandatory ventilation
INH	isoniazid
IPPB	intermittent positive-pressure breathing
I.U.	international units
IV	intravenous or intravenously
IVP	intravenous pyelogram
K, K^+	potassium
kcal	kilocalorie
KCl	potassium chloride
KPO_4	potassium phosphate
KUB	x-ray of abdomen (kidneys, ureters, bowels)
L	liter
LDH	lactate dehydrogenase
LDL	low-density lipoprotein
LLQ	lower left quadrant
LP	lumbar puncture, low potency
LR	lactated Ringer's (solution) (also RL)
lt.	left
M	meter
mA	milliampere
MB	myocardial band (see CPK-MB)
MBC	minimal bacterial concentration
MED	minimum erythema dose
mEq	milliequivalent
mg	milligram
Mg	magnesium
μg	microgram
MI	myocardial infarction
MIC	minimum inhibitory concentration
ml	milliliter
mm	millimeter
MOM	milk of magnesia
MRI	magnetic resonance imaging
Na, Na^+	sodium
$NaHCO_3$	sodium bicarbonate
Neuro	neurologic
NG	nasogastric
NKA	no known allergies
NPH	neutral protamine Hagedorn (insulin)
NPO	nulla per os (nothing by mouth)
NS	normal saline solution (0.9%)
½NS	0.45% saline solution
NSAID	nonsteroidal antiinflammatory drug
O_2	oxygen
Osm	osmolality
OT	occupational therapy
OTC	over the counter
p̄, post	after
PA	posteroanterior; pulmonary artery
Pa_{O_2}	arterial oxygen pressure

P_AO_2, PA_{O_2}	partial pressure of oxygen in alveolar gas
p.c.	post cibum (after meals)
pCO_2, PCO_2	partial pressure of carbon dioxide
PEEP	positive end-expiratory pressure
pH	hydrogen ion concentration (H+)
PID	pelvic inflammatory disease
PO	per os (by mouth)
pO_2, PO_2	partial pressure of oxygen
polys	polymorphonuclear leukocytes
PPD	purified protein derivative
pr	per rectum
prn	pro re nata (as needed)
Pro	prothrombin
PT	physical therapy; prothrombin time
PTCA	percutaneous transluminal coronary angioplasty
PTT	partial thromboplastin time
PVC	premature ventricular contraction
q	quaque (every)
q 6 h, q 2 h	every 6 hours; every 2 hours
qd	quaque die (every day)
q.i.d.	quarter in die (four times a day)
q.o.d.	every other day
RA	rheumatoid arthritis; room air; right atrial
Resp	respiratory rate
RL	Ringer's lactated solution (also LR)
R/O	rule out
ROM	range of motion
rt.	right
s̄	sine (without)
SBP	systolic blood pressure
SC	subcutaneous; subcutaneously
SGOT	serum glutamic-oxaloacetic transaminase (AST)
SGPT	serum glutamic-pyruvic transaminase (ALT)
SIADH	syndrome of inappropriate antidiuretic hormone
sl	sublingually
SLE	systemic lupus erythematosus
SMA-12	sequential multiple analysis; a battery of 12 chemistry tests performed together on a 12-channel autoanalyzer. Tests included vary according to the institution but generally include Na^+, K^+, HCO_3^-, Cl^-, BUN, glucose, creatinine, bilirubin, calcium, total protein, albumin, and alkaline phosphatase. Other chemistry batteries include SMA-6 and SMA-20
SMX	sulfamethoxazole
s/p	status post (the state after; the state of being after, for example, a myocardial infarction)
SSKI	saturated solution of potassium iodide

STAT	statim (immediately—to be done as fast as possible, on an emergency, first priority basis)
susp	suspension
T4, T3RU	thyroxine level (T4) and triiodothyronine resin uptake—a common thyroid screening test combination
tab	tablet
TB	tuberculosis
Temp	temperature
THC	tetrahydrocannabinol
TIA	transient ischemic attack
t.i.d.	ter in die (three times a day)
TKO	to keep open, an infusion rate (usually 500 ml/24h)—just enough to keep the IV from clotting
TMP	trimethoprim
TMP-SMX	trimethoprim-sulfamethoxazole combination
TPA	tissue plasminogen activator
TSH	thyroid-stimulating hormone
TSS	toxic shock syndrome
U	units
UA	urinalysis
URI	upper respiratory infection
UTI	urinary tract infection
UV-B	ultraviolet B light, having a wavelength of 290–320 nm
VAC	vincristine, Adriamycin, and cyclophosphamide
VC	vital capacity
VDRL	Venereal Disease Research Laboratory
VF	ventricular fibrillation
VLDL	very low-density lipoprotein
VPB, VPC	ventricular premature beats or contractions (also PVC)
VS	vital signs
VT	ventricular tachycardia
W	water
WBC	white blood cell, white blood count

NOTE

We have made every responsible effort to include treatments based on current medical practice. The indications, dosages, and side effects are based upon a number of sources. Drug indications and dosages in this book may not, in all cases, be in agreement with recommendations of the Food and Drug Administration. The manufacturer's package insert is the best source of information on FDA approval for dosages and indications. Physicians should consult pharmacologic references (including package inserts) when there is doubt or unfamiliarity with drug dosages, indications, or side effects.

ALL DOSAGES ARE FOR ADULTS ONLY

PART I

ADMITTING ORDERS

PHILOSOPHY OF ADMITTING ORDERS

The secret of caring for the patient is caring for the patient.

FRANCIS W. PEABODY, M.D.
The Care of the Patient, 1927

Dr. Peabody's famous statement is an appropriate beginning for a discussion of admitting orders. The statement reminds us that good order writing by itself is not sufficient for good or even adequate medical care. As Peabody also states, "One of the essential qualities of the clinician is interest in humanity." In caring for patients, "the good physician knows his patients through and through" and dispenses time, sympathy, and understanding to them. In addition, the physician scientifically applies principles of diagnosis and treatment. All this constitutes caring for the patient.

Medical knowledge has grown exponentially in the past several decades, and medical care has become a mosaic of many health professionals providing these skills. The physician is increasingly dependent upon others to care adequately for patients. Patient care would not be possible today without a form of communication such as medical order writing. Order writing is the medium by which physicians convey what they want done in the care of their patients.

Because it is such an integral part of caring for patients, the writing of medical orders demands a systematic approach, which forms the foundation leading to a unique set of orders for each patient. In this sense, order writing is similar to such basic components of patient care as the physical examination, medical history, differential diagnosis, and treatment plan. The approach must be orderly and based on sound principles, and the task must be individually tailored to meet each patient's needs.

The elements of the order writing system are outlined in the next section, "Components of Admitting Orders." Included is a mnemonic device designed to assure that all important elements are contained in a patient's admitting orders. The student and practitioner would do well to adopt this or another system to ensure that a complete set of orders will be provided for their patients.

The diverse elements of medical orders convey information in a variety of ways. Orders such as the *admitting diagnosis, patient condition,* and *allergies* communicate vital information that others caring for or interested in the patient must know. Such information should be as accurate as possible. Unknown or probable information is best identified as such.

Most orders request others to make observations or administer treatments. These orders are best grouped into logical categories (e.g., *Vital Signs, Medications, Laboratory Tests, Intravenous Fluids*). Such grouping allows for clarity and ease of interpretation. In addition, in the modern hospital where orders are commonly sent to other departments (e.g., Pharmacy), ordering by category is simply more efficient.

Orders requesting others to do tasks are best written as specifically and unambiguously as possible. A medication order reading "antibiotics for pneumonia" is obviously inadequate because it is too general. Similarly, "penicillin 500 q 4" and "IVs—D5" are inadequate because they are ambiguous. (These orders were encountered in a review of medical orders at a university teaching hospital.) The complete order generally states when the order was written (date and time), what, how much, how often, how long, and perhaps the indication for the order. In the case of medication or IV orders, a specific, clearly written order contains the name of the drug, dosage or concentration, route of administration, frequency or rate, duration, and indication (e.g., if it is to be given prn, or "as needed"). The rationale for such explicitness is that errors are avoided. Such orders prevent others from having to make decisions that should have been specified by the physician. Furthermore, explicitly written orders allow the ward and hospital to operate more efficiently.

An important aspect of any communication is how it is directed and to whom. Ideally, orders written by the physician display respect and consideration for those who have to read them. Legible handwriting, orders written without heavy-handed authoritarianism, appropriate use of polite phrases such as "please" and "thanks" and, again, a systematic, orderly approach communicate a caring and respectful attitude. In so doing, physicians promote respect for all members of the health care team and encourage concern for and careful treatment of their patients.

COMPONENTS OF ADMITTING ORDERS

Admitting orders contain standard information and instructions that serve to direct patient care throughout hospitalization. For each patient, a unique set of admitting orders reflecting condition and problems is required. In this section, the components that should be a part of each patient's admitting orders are discussed.

Important principles in order writing are completeness and standardization. Each set of orders should contain certain components. The physician needs to establish a framework and build the admitting orders around it. It is useful to memorize the components so that important orders are not omitted. A mnemonic device that we have found helpful, and which has the ring of a Dutch seacaptain's name, is "ADCA VAN DIMLS." The letters in ADCA VAN DIMLS stand for the following components of admitting orders:

A– Admission Order
D– Diagnosis
C– Condition
A– Allergies

V– Vital Signs
A– Activity
N– Nursing

D– Diet
I – IV Orders
M–Medication Orders
L– Laboratory Studies
S– Special Orders

If this mnemonic device (or an equivalent one) is used to guide order writing, there is little likelihood that oversights or forgetfulness will prevent patients from receiving important medical treatment or evaluation.

The format used in discussing the components of admitting orders will be the same as that used in all subsequent sections dealing with specific admitting orders. In the left column the specific orders will be written exactly as they might appear in an order book. The right column describes important features of the order and discusses the rationale, exceptions, and problems associated with the specific order.

The following is an example of standard admitting orders with a discussion of the various components.

Example
9/4/93*
2100 hours

1. Admit to Medicine, 5 South

1. The admission order begins each set of admitting orders and states to which service or location the patient has been admitted. After the admission order has been written, the nursing staff can begin to record and act on the subsequent orders.

2. Diagnosis: Pneumonia

2. The diagnosis states the diagnosis or symptom that led to the patient's admission. The diagnosis should be as specific as possible. For example, an admitting diagnosis on our sample patient might read "fever, productive cough, rule out pneumonia" if the diagnosis were not known. Or, the same patient might be described as having *"Hemophilus influenzae* pneumonia, right middle lobe." If a patient has a complication or unique feature to the admitting diagnosis, this should be stated. For example, *"H. influenzae* pneumonia, respiratory failure" would be stated for the patient with severe pneumonia requiring intubation.

2a. Diagnosis: Pneumonia
2°: Chronic obstructive lung disease, Type II diabetes mellitus

2a. Secondary diagnoses can also be given with the primary admitting diagnosis. For example, an elderly patient with pneumonia, chronic obstructive lung disease, and diabetes mellitus would be given admitting diagnoses as noted.

*All orders should be dated, with the hour noted. In the specific admitting orders that follow in this manual, we have elected to exclude the date and time of the order, as it serves no purpose in the context of our book.

The diagnosis is used by the nursing staff to formulate a nursing care plan. It usually appears on medication and nursing worksheets. Because the diagnosis remains with the patient, care must be taken to provide an accurate one. In some hospitals, the diagnosis written on the order sheet is used by administration personnel to keep statistics on hospital admissions.

3. Condition: Serious

3. The condition of the patient on admission is routinely noted. Most hospitals have predefined conditions, such as *satisfactory, serious,* and *critical.* This information is often what is told to families and, on rare occasions, to the media. In addition, some hospitals use the designated condition as a basis for allocating nursing staff. Most importantly, it can be used as a guide by the nursing staff in devising appropriate staffing levels.

A *satisfactory* condition implies that a patient's condition is stable or improving and that a relatively low level of nursing care is required. Patients admitted for minor illnesses or routine elective surgery or procedures are usually classified in this manner.

The designation *serious* means that a patient has a potentially life-threatening or morbid illness with a deteriorating or uncertain course. Nursing care demands are heavier. Most patients with urgent or emergency admissions fall into this category.

The term *critical* applies to those extremely ill patients who are in grave danger of dying. These patients usually demand the highest level of nursing care. Virtually all intensive care unit patients are in "critical" condition.

4. Allergies: Codeine

4. Any medication allergies should be recorded. Ideally, the nature of the reaction should be noted as well. For example, different types of penicillin allergy might be written:

    Penicillin—skin rash, delayed

    Penicillin—urticaria, laryngospasm, immediate

    This information will be noted on the medication "Kardex" used by the nursing staff and will be highlighted on the chart. Pharmacists also use allergy information when comparing the patient's drug profile with a new medication order.

5. Vital Signs: BP, Pulse, Temp, Resp q 4 h
   Call physician if:
   BP < 90/50
   Pulse > 120
   Resp > 25
   Temp > 38.5° C
   Or for any other sudden change in vital signs

5. Vital signs routinely include measurements of blood pressure, pulse rate, temperature, and respiratory rate. The order should state which signs are to be measured and how frequently. Many physicians simply write "routine"; this practice should be avoided since the meaning of "routine" may vary according to the floor or type of patient.

    How often vital signs are taken should be evaluated periodically. Usually, if a patient is improving, vital signs can be taken less often; the patient is therefore disturbed less, allowing for more rest. (This is especially important in elderly patients, who may become confused with frequent disturbances.) An appropriate vital signs order would be: Vital Signs: BP, Pulse, Temp, Resp q 6 h when awake, but at least 3 ×/day. Such an order assures that the patient is seen three times per day and has a night's uninterrupted sleep.

    It is sometimes useful, particularly in unstable clinical situations, to establish boundaries on vital signs and to make a request to be called if the readings fall below or exceed the boundaries. One- or two-sided limits can be given. In the example provided, only one-sided limits were used. Examples of two-sided limits are: Call physician if:

Systolic BP < 90 or > 200
Diastolic BP < 50 or > 100
Pulse < 50 or > 120
Resp < 8 or > 25

Failure to establish acceptable variations in vital sign measurements can result in confusion and undetected deterioration in the patient's clinical status. Standing orders or written policies are helpful but are not specific enough for all patients. The nature of the vital sign orders will depend upon the clinical setting and type of hospital. For example, in critical care units it is usually sufficient to write "Vital Signs: as deemed necessary." In hospitals that use primary nursing (care provided primarily by registered nurses), the nurses can assume responsibility for deciding how often determination of vital signs is necessary. The physician can write "Vital Signs: at least q 6 h for 24 h, then as deemed necessary."

6. Activity: Bed rest with bathroom privileges

6. For patients who require no restriction of activity, one usually writes "ad lib." This order implies that a patient may do whatever he or she desires short of leaving the floor. Permission to leave the medical floor or hospital is usually stated under Activity.

The level of activity ranges from "ad lib" to "complete bed rest." Between these two extremes are a variety of other levels of activity, e.g., bed rest, up in a chair t.i.d.; bed rest, ambulate in hall b.i.d.; bed rest, commode privileges. In primary nursing settings, these decisions can be made by the nursing staff. This order will be changed frequently, depending on the patient's condition. Activity status should be reviewed and revised as needed.

7. Nursing:
   Daily weights
   I and O
   Incentive spirometry
   Encourage deep breathing and coughing
   Measure blood glucose with "Chemstrips" 9 AM (fasting) and 9 PM (2100 h) and chart results

7. This section specifies what the nursing staff is to do for the patient. In the example of a patient with pneumonia who is receiving intravenous fluids, the physician writes an order that the patient be weighed daily and that intake and output be measured and recorded. I and O should be charted for all patients receiving IV fluids.

   In addition, the nurses are asked to provide the patient with an incentive spirometer and to encourage the patient to breathe deeply and cough.

   Since this patient is diabetic, the nurses are asked to measure the blood sugar at the bedside using automatic lancet and a glucose oxidase–impregnated plastic strip (Chemstrip). In acutely ill patients with diabetes, blood glucose monitoring should be more intensive since they frequently develop symptomatic hyperglycemia due to stress.

8. Diet: 1500-calorie diabetic diet
   Encourage fluids

8. The diet order prescribes the diet the patient will have. Diets range from "house," or "regular," which means that the patient will select choices from the hospital menu, to "NPO," meaning that the patient receives nothing by mouth. Diets are prescribed on the basis of: (1) Sodium content—e.g., 2 g sodium is a common diet prescription for a patient with congestive heart failure. (2) Protein content—e.g., persons with renal or hepatic failure may have protein restricted to perhaps 60 g per day. (3) Calories—in this example, the patient will receive only 1500 calories, as recommended by the American Diabetic Association.

Weight-reduction diets usually contain a caloric restriction. (4) Fat content—patients who are being observed for malabsorption may be placed on a diet of 100 g of fat per day. More commonly, fat and cholesterol are restricted. (5) Consistency of food—postoperative patients or those with gastrointestinal disease may gradually advance from clear to full liquids, to puréed or soft solids, to a house diet. (6) Types of foods—most hospitals have a variety of diets by food type. For example, hospitals may offer high-residue diets for patients with diverticulosis or irritable bowel syndrome. Other diets available include low-residue, bland, gluten-free, and lactose-free.

The diet order can also contain instruction about fluids allowed by mouth. The physician in this example has requested that fluids be "pushed," which means that the nursing and dietary staffs should encourage the patient to drink as much as possible. The order also implies that liquids should be available at the patient's bedside. Conversely, the patient with cirrhosis and ascites probably requires fluid restriction, e.g., "1000 ml fluid restriction."

9. IV Orders:
   #1. 1000 ml NS at 125 ml/h
   #2. 1000 ml ½NS at 125 ml/h
   #3. 1000 ml ½NS at 50 ml/h

9. In general, intravenous orders should be written for a 24-h period only. The order should state the type of solution to be infused, how much, and at what rate. Ideally, each IV bottle should be numbered sequentially throughout the hospitalization. For continuous infusion of the same solution, the duration of the infusion and a stop order should be written.

Intravenous solutions often contain additives such as potassium chloride, sodium bicarbonate, or multiple vitamin mixtures. For example, "1000 ml D5NS with 20 mEq KCl at 125 ml/h over 8 h" is a commonly used combination. Orders for blood products (packed cells, plasma, platelets) and other IV substances are also written in this section. For patients with more than one IV, separate orders must be written, stating clearly the use of each.

When patients require intravenous access for medication only, an IV order must still be written. Usually, the IV is put to a "heparin lock," which means that it is flushed with heparin, 10 units, and normal saline, 10 ml, every 6–8 h. Heparin comes in standard "Tubex" form, and the volume and concentration need not be specified unless patient needs dictate otherwise. (Some hospitals still use 100-unit Tubex.)

The IV may also be connected to a solution, which is infused at a slow rate to keep open (TKO) the vein, written "500 ml D5W, TKO over 24 h."

10. Medications:
    Ampicillin 1 g IV q 6 h
    NPH insulin 15 units SC q AM
    Routine: Triazolam 0.25 mg PO q hs prn sleep, may repeat × 1
    Milk of magnesia (MOM) 30 ml PO q hs prn if no stool that day
    Dioctyl sodium sulfosuccinate (DOSS) 250 mg PO every day
    Acetaminophen 650 mg PO q 4 h prn for Temp > 38° C or pain

10. Medication orders contain the name of the drug (generic name preferred), the amount (dose) desired, and the route and the frequency or time of administration. The duration of administration may also be given. "As needed," or prn, orders should always specify the indication.

It is preferable to begin medication orders with drugs for a specific therapeutic purpose—in this case, an antibiotic likely to be effective for the patient's presumed *H. influenzae* pneumonia and insulin for diabetes. Next, the orders for routine medications and symptomatic treatment are given. Most patients have some difficulty sleeping in a hospital environment; routinely ordering a hypnotic is helpful. A variety of hypnotics are available and effective for short-term use; the specific hypnotic should be chosen carefully, and thus different hypnotics will be ordered in the specific admitting orders that follow in this manual. Bed rest often results in constipation; therefore, most patients are provided with an order for stool softeners or a gentle cathartic as needed. In this example, the physician has anticipated that the patient may need an antipyretic and analgesic medication and has ordered acetaminophen as needed. Careful anticipation of the patient's routine medication needs will prevent late-night phone calls and the need to page the physician. Other routine symptomatic medications include sedatives, antiemetics, antidiarrheal agents, and narcotic analgesics. The ordering of medications must be done judiciously, since these orders increase nursing and pharmacy workloads and, if excessive, may be quite costly.

Medication orders should be written with great care. Many medications are commonly prescribed for hospitalized patients, of whom a disturbingly high percentage suffer from side effects. For this reason, many hospitals require that medication orders be renewed at intervals, usually weekly. This requirement is useful since it sets a standard time for the reassessment of medication orders. In addition, since medications are added during the course of a hospitalization, rewriting orders periodically provides an opportunity to review the medications a patient is receiving and to consider potential drug interactions.

11. Laboratory:
    Admission: CBC, UA, SMA-12, CXR, blood cultures (2), sputum Gram stain and culture—done
    Tonight: ECG, save for physician
    Tomorrow AM: Hct, WBC, fasting glucose, electrolytes, sputum for TB stain and culture

11. Orders for laboratory studies are usually written in a separate section. It is preferable to list laboratory studies already performed as part of the admitting orders. This allows the nurses to know what studies have been done. In addition, the covering house staff who have not written orders for the patient can see what work has been done and thus will not needlessly duplicate laboratory studies.

    Laboratory studies for the next 24 h should be ordered, e.g., "Sputum for TB (or AFB) stain and culture $\times$ 3; AM sputum samples." In general, routine laboratory studies should be avoided, since they result in needless expense and blood loss.

    Ideally, requisitions and consultation forms should be completed by the physician making the request for laboratory studies. If the physician does not fill out x-ray, nuclear medicine, or other requisitions, orders for these studies should contain a statement about the indication, clinical summary, or suspected diagnosis. This information can then be transcribed by the ward clerk and transmitted to the radiologist who is responsible for performing and interpreting the x-ray or diagnostic study. Although it is not ideal, we have adopted this format in our book.

12. Special: Respiratory therapy t.i.d. for cough, and percussion and drainage (right middle lobe pneumonia, COPD)

12. Special orders include ancillary services (respiratory, physical, or occupational therapy), consultations, special preparations for diagnostic studies, and any other orders that do not conveniently fit into the other categories. Special equipment (e.g., a bed board) and precautions (e.g., isolation procedures, a light beside the bed to lessen con-

fusion) can also be included in this category. However, verbal communication between the doctor and the nurse on rounds may be a better way to accomplish these aspects of patient care.

Thank you,

_____
(Physician's signature)

_____ M.D.
(Printed name)

All orders must close with a legible signature. In a teaching hospital with a rotating house staff, the signer will note his or her position and service. We recommend printing one's name (or using a stamp) under the signature. Unsigned and illegible orders can cause excess work, especially for nurses and pharmacists, who not only must try to decipher the order's content but also may need to use detective-like skills to identify and find the writer if clarification of an order is required.

A "thank you" is an important closing touch. Taking the time to express appreciation generates a congenial atmosphere and enhances the self-respect of all who pursue the demanding job of caring for sick persons.

PART II

SPECIFIC ADMITTING ORDERS

CARDIOVASCULAR DISEASE

ARRHYTHMIAS

It is difficult to anticipate the many cardiac arrhythmias that occur in cardiovascular disease, and hence it is laborious to write admitting orders to cover all the rhythms likely to require immediate therapy. In many coronary and intensive care units, standing orders exist to facilitate arrhythmia therapy. It is assumed that the standing orders will be followed by the nursing staff unless a statement is made to the contrary in the admitting orders. Of course, if the hospital does not have standing orders, the appropriate orders must be written upon admission or during the course of hospitalization. In this section, standing orders for several arrhythmias are listed.

All patients likely to require therapy for arrhythmias should have cardiac rhythm monitored continuously and a reliable IV or heparin lock in place.

Asystole

1. Call a cardiac arrest code.
2. If a pacemaker is in place, begin ventricular pacing on the demand mode at a rate of 75/min and an amplitude of 10 mA.
3. If there is no response, begin CPR and give epinephrine (1:10,000) 1 mg IV push. May repeat in 5 min.
4. If no response, give atropine 1 mg IV push.

Bradycardia

1. Heart rate below 60: Notify the physician on call.
2. Heart rate below 50: If pacemaker wires or catheter is in place, begin ventricular pacing on the demand mode at a rate of 75/min and notify the physician on call.
3. If the heart rate is below 40 or the patient is symptomatic with a heart rate below 50, give atropine 0.5 mg IV and notify the physician on call.

Heart Block—Third Degree A-V Block

1. Notify the physician on call. For patients with deteriorating vital signs, begin the treatment listed below.
2. If pacemaker wires or catheter is in place, begin ventricular pacing on the demand mode at a rate of 75/min and an amplitude of 10 mA.
3. If there is no pacemaker, give atropine 0.5 mg IV.
4. Be prepared to initiate external massage.

Ventricular Fibrillation (VF)

1. Perform a precordial thump only if arrest was witnessed.
2. Defibrillate 200 joules as soon as possible. Begin CPR if there is a delay in defibrillation.

3. If VF persists, immediately defibrillate 200–300 joules.
4. If VF persists, immediately defibrillate up to 360 joules.
5. Begin CPR if defibrillatory shocks are unsuccessful.
6. Give epinephrine (1:10,000) 0.5 mg IV push.
7. Defibrillate up to 360 joules.
8. Give lidocaine 1 mg/kg IV push, and repeat defibrillatory shock (up to 360 joules) for persistent VF.
9. If defibrillation occurs, begin a lidocaine drip 2 mg/min IV.

Ventricular Tachycardia (VT) or Flutter

1. No pulse. Therapy is the same as for ventricular fibrillation.
2. Pulse present and stable:
   a. Give lidocaine 1 mg/kg IV push.
   b. If VT persists, repeat lidocaine every 5–10 min 0.5 mg/kg IV push up to 3 mg/kg.
   c. If VT converts, start a lidocaine drip—2 mg/min IV.
3. Pulse present and unstable:
   a. If vital signs are deteriorating, cardiovert at 50 joules. If patient is conscious, sedation with midazolam (1–5 mg IV) may be used cautiously.
   b. If unsuccessful, cardiovert at 100 joules, 200 joules, and up to 360 joules.
   c. If unsuccessful, give lidocaine 1 mg/kg IV, then repeat cardioversion at 360 joules.
   d. If VT converts, start a lidocaine drip 2 mg/min IV.

CARDIOGENIC SHOCK

1. Admit to CCU

1. Optimal therapy for cardiogenic shock requires a critical care facility capable of determining pulmonary capillary wedge pressure and monitoring arterial pressure.

2. Diagnosis: Cardiogenic shock

2. The definition of cardiogenic shock varies, but it generally refers to hypotension with insufficient organ perfusion as a result of cardiac pathology (usually acute myocardial infarction).

3. Condition: Critical

3. The mortality rate from cardiogenic shock is over 90%.

4. Allergies: No known allergies

4. Routine, may be abbreviated NKA.

5. Vital Signs: As deemed necessary; continuous arterial pressure monitoring
   Call physician if:
   BP <60 systolic

5. Many CCUs have standard vital sign monitoring. It is not necessary to write specific orders in a setting where vital signs may change so fre-

Resp >30
Pulse >120
Temp >38.5°C

6. Activity: Strict bed rest

7. Nursing:
I and O
Daily weights
O₂ 4 L/min by nasal cannula
Swan-Ganz and arterial pressure line care
Foley catheter

8. Diet: NPO except for sips of water

9. IV Orders:
#1. 500 ml D5W TKO
#2. Maintain arterial line with continuous heparin flush system
#3. Maintain Swan-Ganz line with continuous heparin flush system

10. Medications:
Morphine 1–5 mg IV q 30 min prn for pain or restlessness
Dopamine—start at 3 μg/kg/min IV and titrate to optimize blood pressure and cardiac output

11. Laboratory:
Admission: STAT electrolytes, BUN, and glucose; SMA-12, CBC, UA, CPK and CPK-MB, ECG, portable CXR
Tomorrow: ECG, SMA-12

quently. It is the job of the CCU nurse to monitor vital signs as frequently as the patient's condition warrants.

6. Routine.

7. Patients with obstructive lung disease should initially receive no more than 2 L/min of oxygen unless severe hypoxia is present. Most CCUs have routine care for Swan-Ganz and arterial pressure lines. Patients will usually require Foley catheterization to measure urine output accurately.

8. Patients with mild hypotension may be alert enough for a 2 g Na diet.

9. Most CCUs have routines for maintaining a continuous heparin flush system.

10. Dopamine, or dobutamine, is indicated as the initial inotropic agent when volume status is adequate. Unloading therapy, using nitroprusside, nitroglycerine, or amrinone may be indicated for low cardiac output states when there is increased systemic vascular resistance. For selected patients, the use of intraaortic balloon counterpulsation may be necessary.

11. The heart-specific creatine phosphokinase (CPK-MB) provides a fast and sensitive way of diagnosing a myocardial infarction (MI). It is almost always elevated within 18 hours of symptoms. If symptoms preceded admission by more than 36 hours, measurement of LDH and its isoenzymes may provide biochemical confirmation of infarction.

12. Special: None

12. One should consider the need for urgent cardiac catheterization or echocardiography to define potentially treatable cardiac conditions in the setting of clearcut myocardial infarction (based on history and ECG). Thrombolytic agents may be useful if onset is ≤6 h prior to time of therapy. (See pp. 188–189.)

CONGESTIVE HEART FAILURE (CHF)

1. Admit to 5 North

1. Mild CHF occurring in a patient with a remote chance of having an acute MI can be managed on a general medical ward, but more severe cases should be admitted to an intensive care or coronary care unit.

2. Diagnosis: Congestive heart failure

2. The possibility of an MI precipitating the CHF necessitates "R/O MI" studies and precautions.

3. Condition: Serious

3. The most typical patient condition is "serious." Severe CHF should be listed as "critical."

4. Allergies: NKA

4. Routine.

5. Vital Signs: Pulse, Resp, BP q 2 h × 4, then q 4 h × 6, then q shift; Temp q shift
Call physician if:
BP >160 systolic
<80 systolic
Resp >30
Pulse >120
Temp >38.5°C

5. For patients admitted to an ICU, it is often sufficient to write "as deemed necessary," since it is the responsibility of the ICU nurse to monitor vital signs as frequently as the patient's condition warrants.

6. Activity: Bed rest with commode for 24 h, then up as tolerated

6. Bed rest facilitates diuresis.

7. Nursing:
Daily weights
I and O
Elevate head of bed 30–45°
O₂ 2 L/min by nasal cannula

7. Daily weights are a reliable method of determining the adequacy of diuresis. I and O should be measured in critically ill patients until their condition stabilizes. Discontinuing an I and O order when it is no longer needed will free the staff for more im-

portant tasks. Patients with more serious CHF may require higher FiO_2.

8. Diet: 2 g Na

8. Sodium restriction promotes diuresis and inhibits further fluid accumulation.

9. IV Orders: Heparin lock

9. Patients with more serious CHF should have 500 ml D5W TKO continued for 24 h or until stable.

10. Medications:
    Furosemide 20 mg IV now
    Digoxin 0.5 mg IV now
    Routine:
    DOSS 250 mg PO every day
    MOM 30 ml PO q hs prn
    Triazolam 0.25 mg PO q hs prn for sleep; may repeat once

10. Patients already taking furosemide should receive twice their usual daily dose. The regimen for IV and oral digitalization is outlined under "Cardiovascular Therapeutic Agents." Patients who present a clinical picture with pulmonary edema should receive aggressive therapy such as morphine sulfate, 4 mg IV, STAT; furosemide, 40 mg IV STAT.

11. Laboratory:
    Admission: STAT: Electrolytes, BUN, glucose; CBC, UA, portable CXR; ECG
    Tomorrow: SMA-12

11. Determining the K+ level is important for patients on digitalis and diuretics. Patients on a R/O MI protocol should have the appropriate laboratory tests ordered. (See the section on "Myocardial Infarction.") Severely ill patients should be followed with ABGs.

12. Special: None

12. As indicated.

DISSECTING THORACIC AORTIC ANEURYSM

1. Admit to ICU

1. Optimal therapy for dissecting aortic aneurysm requires close monitoring of arterial pressure and clinical status.

2. Diagnosis:
   Dissecting thoracic aortic aneurysm

2. Dissection of the aorta can occur in the ascending portion with antegrade propagation beyond the arch (Type I), limited to the ascending thoracic aorta (Type II), or limited to the descending thoracic aorta (Type III) or with retrograde

spread from the descending aorta back around the arch. Most commonly, dissection occurs at a site of aneurysmal dilatation or decreased wall strength due to connective tissue disease.

3. Condition: Critical

3. Untreated aortic dissection has a mortality rate of over 25% at 24 h.

4. Allergies: NKA

4. Routine.

5. Vital Signs: As deemed necessary; continuous arterial pressure monitoring
   Call physician if:
   Systolic BP >120 or < 70
   Pulse > 120
   Resp > 30
   Temp > 38.5°C
   Call physician if sudden (> 30 mm Hg) drop in systolic BP, and stop nitroprusside drip

5. Most ICUs have standard vital sign monitoring. It is the job of the ICU nurse to monitor vital signs as frequently as the patient's condition warrants. Measurement of moment-to-moment changes in blood pressure and heart rate is essential, usually by use of continuous ECG monitoring and peripheral arterial line.

6. Activity: Strict bed rest, environmental noise and activity kept to a minimum (aneurysm precautions)

6. Decreased stimulation of the patient will help reduce heart rate, blood pressure, and catecholamine release.

7. Nursing:
   I and O
   O$_2$ 2 L/min by nasal cannula
   Foley catheter care
   Arterial pressure line and Swan-Ganz catheter care

7. Patients will usually require close monitoring of urine output, direct measurement of arterial pressure, and often measurement of cardiac filling and performance. Most ICUs have routine care for arterial lines and Swan-Ganz catheters.

8. Diet: NPO; may have ice chips, glycerin swabs for dry mouth

8. Depending on the site of dissection and compromise of vital organs, patients may require immediate emergency angiography or surgery.

9. IV Orders:
   #1. 500 ml D5W TKO
   #2. Maintain arterial line with continuous heparin flush system
   #3. Maintain Swan-Ganz line with continuous heparin flush system

9. Most ICUs have routines for maintaining continuous heparin flush systems.

10. Medications:
    Morphine 1–5 mg IV q 30 min prn for pain or restlessness
    Nitroprusside 50 mg in 250 ml D5W; start at 0.03

10. The major goal of therapy is to rapidly reduce aortic wall stress by decreasing heart rate and blood pressure. Pain, often severe, is present in up

mg/min IV and titrate to systolic BP 100–120 mm Hg or lowest level consistent with adequate organ perfusion

Propranolol 1 mg IV over 5 min and repeat until pulse < 60 or to a total dose of 0.15 mg/kg. Repeat dose every 4–6 hours

to 90% of patients and contributes to increased sympathetic tone. A physician should be at hand during initial infusion of nitroprusside and propranolol until stable low blood pressure has been achieved.

11. Laboratory:
Admission: Electrolytes, BUN, creatinine, glucose, CBC, PT and PTT, STAT; UA; portable CXR, ECG, STAT. Type and crossmatch 4 units whole blood, 6 units packed red blood cells, STAT

Tomorrow: CBC, electrolytes, BUN, creatinine, glucose, portable CXR, ECG. Thiocyanate level (if continued on nitroprusside)

11. Treatment and data gathering should be done as quickly and unobtrusively as possible. Adequate amounts of blood products must be available, especially if surgery is anticipated. Potentially toxic levels of thiocyanate can accumulate after 24–48 hours of nitroprusside infusion.

12. Special:
A. Echocardiography, STAT
B. Cardiac surgeon consulted and may write preop orders

12. Rapid diagnosis and confirmation of anatomy are essential in planning appropriate surgical or medical management. The imaging procedure of choice will vary based on timing and availability of equipment and personnel. Transesophageal echocardiography, CT scanning, magnetic resonance imaging (MRI), and angiography can all provide useful diagnostic and anatomic information and may be used singly or in combination. In most cases, thoracic or cardiac surgeons are closely involved throughout the course, especially at the onset.

HYPERTENSIVE CRISIS

1. Admit to ICU

1. Arterial line monitoring should be done.

2. Diagnosis: Hypertensive crisis

2. Hypertensive crisis means a life-threatening surge in blood pressure. Other associated clinical findings include pulmonary edema, encepha-

lopathy, angina, myocardial infarction, retinal hemorrhage and papilledema, proteinuria, and renal failure.

3. Condition: Critical

3. Self-explanatory.

4. Allergies: NKA

4. Routine.

5. Vital Signs: Continuous arterial pressure monitoring, BP, Resp, Pulse q 15 min × 4, then q 30 min × 4, then q 1 h × 4, then q 2 h × 4, then q 4 h; Temp q shift

5. For ICU patients, it is often sufficient to write "as deemed necessary," since it is the responsibility of the ICU nurse to monitor vital signs as frequently as the patient's condition warrants.

6. Activity: Strict bed rest

6. Routine.

7. Nursing:
I and O
Daily weights
Neuro check q 1 h × 8, then q 4 h
O$_2$ 2 L/min by nasal cannula

7. Routine.

8. Diet: NPO × 24 h except for ice chips

8. Routine.

9. IV Orders: 500 ml D5W TKO; maintain arterial line with continuous heparin flush system.

9. The use of saline should be avoided for the first 24 h, and then maintenance fluids can be started cautiously. IV potassium supplements may be required, depending on the serum level.

10. Medications:
Nitroprusside 50 mg in 250 ml D5W; start at 0.03 mg/min IV—titrate to BP (a systolic of 140–170 and a diastolic of 100–110); do not exceed 0.5 mg/min

10. Initiation of a nitroprusside drip requires a physician to titrate the dose until reasonably stable blood pressures are achieved. Depending on the severity of the clinical situation, other drugs may be used. Nifedipine 10 mg sublingually is another easy, safe, and rapidly effective (10–15 min) way to reduce BP and thus is an attractive option.

11. Laboratory:
Admission: Electrolytes, CBC, creatinine, BUN, glucose, STAT; UA; portable CXR, ECG, STAT
Tomorrow: SMA-12

11. Treatment and data gathering should be done simultaneously and as quickly as possible.

12. Special: Call physician for sudden fall in blood pressure (> 30 mm Hg systolic), and stop nitroprusside drip

12. This order could also appear under "Medications."

MYOCARDIAL INFARCTION/RULE OUT MYOCARDIAL INFARCTION

1. Admit to CCU

   1. This is routine in the United States. In some other countries, ward and home care may be used for patients with an uncomplicated MI.

2. Diagnosis: R/O myocardial infarction

   2. From a management point of view, there is no distinction between admitting orders for patients admitted to rule out infarctions and those whose diagnosis is a virtual certainty. However, once the diagnosis is confirmed or ruled out, subsequent orders differ considerably. If the likelihood of MI is high (typical history and ECG changes), the diagnosis should be listed as a probable MI.

3. Condition: Serious

   3. "Serious" is the usual condition. Patients in shock or with pulmonary edema should be listed as "critical."

4. Allergies: NKA

   4. Routine.

5. Vital Signs: BP, Pulse, Resp q 4 h and Temp q 8 h for 24 h; then q 6 h if stable
   Call physician if:
   BP <90, >160 systolic
   <60, >110 diastolic
   Pulse >120 or <60
   Resp >25 or <10
   Temp >38.5°C
   Or for any sudden change in vital signs

   5. Many CCUs have standard procedures for taking vital signs. It may be sufficient to write "as deemed necessary," since it is the responsibility of the CCU nurse to monitor vital signs as frequently as the patient's condition warrants.

6. Activity: Bed rest with commode privileges

   6. Patients in more critical condition should probably be on strict bed rest. In some units, all patients are on bed rest precautions.

7. Nursing:
   Daily weights
   I and O
   O_2 2 L/min by nasal cannula
   Continuous ECG monitoring

   7. Measuring I and O may not be necessary if the patient has a heparin lock, is eating adequately, and does not need diuretics.

8. Diet: 1200 calories in 3–4 portions, low fat, no extremes of temperature

   8. Clear liquids are given for the first 24 hours to ease digestion and minimize the likelihood of vomiting. Avoid salt

9. IV Orders: 1000 ml D5W TKO over 48 h

10. Medications:
   Analgesia: Morphine 5 mg IV; may give additional 2 mg IV doses at 5-min intervals to a total of 15 mg if BP and Resp are stable
   Anxiety: Lorazepam 2 mg PO q 6 h
   Hypertension: Nitropaste 2% ointment 1.5 inches q 4–6 h
   Tachycardia (with normal BP): Propranolol 20 mg PO q 6–12 h

11. Laboratory:
   Admission: Electrolytes, BUN, glucose, STAT; UA, CBC, CPK and CPK-MB now—repeat in 6 h; portable CXR
   Tomorrow: SMA-12, ECG

substitutes (KCl) if hyperkalemia is present.

9. The TKO IV is in place for emergency medications.

10. Meperidine is an equally effective IV analgesic. The usual dose is 50 mg IV; additional doses of 20 mg IV may be given at 5-min intervals to a total of 150 mg if BP and Resp are stable. Most MI patients are anxious and benefit from short-term sedation while in the hospital. Reduction of blood pressure and heart rate to low normal values will probably help reduce myocardial oxygen demand.

   In some centers, prophylactic lidocaine is used in the case of an acute MI. In this setting, lidocaine would be given as noted under "Arrhythmias" (see p. 17). In some patients, rapid restoration of coronary blood flow through an area of thrombosis can be achieved with intravenous or intracoronary streptokinase or TPA (tissue plasminogen activator) or by percutaneous transluminal coronary angioplasty (PTCA). These approaches are most likely to be helpful early in the course of infarction ($\leq$ 6 hours from onset of symptoms). They are described in more detail in Part III, "Orders Accompanying Procedures," pp. 188–189.

11. Physicians choosing to anticoagulate their patients should obtain the appropriate clotting studies. The use of isoenzymes to diagnose myocardial damage varies in different locations. The most efficient method is to determine the CPK-MB level on admission and again after 6–12 hours as determined by onset and course of pain. If both are normal, the likelihood of an acute MI diagnosis is slight in

patients admitted soon after having acute symptoms. When the duration of symptoms is longer, or the time of the suspected infarction is unclear, the slower-rising cardiac enzymes (LDH and its isoenzymes) are useful for diagnosis.

In selected patients, cardiac catheterization may be useful during the hospital course to attempt thrombolysis, for possible angioplasty or surgery, or to otherwise determine therapy and prognosis. (See Part III, "Orders Accompanying Procedures.") Standing orders exist in almost all CCUs and should be authorized in the patient's orders.

12. Special: Bed board, antiembolism stockings; standing orders as per routine

12. Routine in some centers.

PULMONARY EMBOLISM

1. Admit to 4 North

1. Patients in whom the chance of pulmonary embolus is remote can be managed on a medical floor while undergoing further diagnostic studies. Those with hypotension or significant hypoxia should be admitted to an intensive care unit.

2. Diagnosis: Pulmonary embolus

2. Patients are often admitted before a definite diagnosis is reached, and "rule out pulmonary embolus" is a common admitting diagnosis.

3. Condition: Serious

3. The condition of the patient may range from satisfactory to critical.

4. Allergies: NKA

4. Routine.

5. Vital Signs: BP, Pulse, Resp q 1 h × 4, then q 2 h × 4, then q 6 h; Temp q 6 h
Call physician if:
BP > 160, < 80 systolic
> 115, < 60 diastolic

5. For patients admitted to an intensive care unit, it is often sufficient to write "as deemed necessary," since it is the responsibility of the nurse to monitor vital signs as fre-

Resp > 30
Pulse > 120

6. Activity: Bed rest with bedside commode

6. Routine.

7. Nursing:
Guaiac all stools
Dipstick urine for blood
O_2 2 L/min by nasal cannula
No intramuscular injections

7. Stools should be checked for occult blood before and during anticoagulation therapy. Patients with more severe hypoxia and respiratory distress may require higher oxygen levels.

8. Diet: As tolerated

8. Critically ill patients should be NPO.

9. IV Orders: See "Medications"

9. See "Medications."

10. Medications:
Heparin 7000 units IV bolus now
Heparin infusion—25,000 units in 500 ml D5W (50 units/ml) beginning at 1000 units/h (to be adjusted to maintain the PTT 1.5–2 × control [INR 2.0–3.0])
Routine:
DOSS 250 mg PO every day
MOM 30 ml PO q hs prn for constipation or no stool that day
Triazolam 0.25 mg PO q hs prn for sleep.

10. Heparin may be given intermittently or continuously. With continuous infusions, a bolus (usually 100 units/kg) is given, followed by an infusion of 20,000–30,000 units/day. Some physicians routinely give antacids to patients on anticoagulants. In patients with right heart failure or more serious pulmonary embolus, thrombolytic therapy with streptokinase, TPA, or urokinase should be considered.

11. Laboratory:
Admission: PTT prior to giving heparin and 4 h after infusion, then every day; PT, electrolytes, BUN, glucose, ABGs, CBC including platelet count, STAT; UA, ECG, CXR (PA and lateral)
Tomorrow: CBC and platelet count, SMA-12

11. There are several methods of monitoring the intrinsic clotting pathway. Usually, a recalcification time or partial thromboplastin time (PTT) is used. The therapeutic range is 1.5–2.0 × control value for the PTT (INR 2.0–3.0) and 225–275 sec for the recalcification time in most U.S. clinical labs. Dose adjustment can be made by physicians or nurses.

12. Special: Lung scan for possible pulmonary embolus, bed board, antiembolism stockings

12. If available, a ventilation perfusion scan is useful in interpreting equivocal findings on a perfusion scan and is frequently ordered as a standard diagnostic study. In equivocal cases or in certain critical settings, a pulmonary angiogram will be useful.

DEEP VENOUS THROMBOSIS

1. Admit to 2 North

   1. Patients can usually be admitted to general medical floors.

2. Diagnosis: Deep venous thrombosis

   2. Therapeutically, deep venous thrombosis is managed similarly to pulmonary embolus.

3. Condition: Satisfactory

   3. The condition of the patient can range from satisfactory to serious.

4. Allergies: NKA

   4. Routine.

5. Vital Signs: q shift

   5. Unless pulmonary embolus is being considered, q shift is sufficient.

6. Activity: Strict bed rest × 24 h

   6. Routine.

7. Nursing:
   Guaiac all stools
   Dipstick urine for blood
   Elevate right leg; warm packs to areas of inflammation b.i.d.

   7. The affected extremity should be elevated. This and the application of heat may provide good symptomatic relief.

8. Diet: See "Pulmonary Embolism"

   8. See "Pulmonary Embolism."

9. IV Orders: See "Medications"

   9. See "Medications."

10. Medications:
    Heparin 7000 units IV bolus now
    Heparin infusion—25,000 units in 500 ml D5W (50 units/ml) beginning at 1000 units/h (to be adjusted to maintain the PTT from 1.5–2.0 × control [INR 2.0–3.0])
    Routine:
    DOSS 250 mg PO every day
    MOM 30 ml PO q hs prn for constipation or no stool that day
    Triazolam 0.25 mg PO q hs prn for sleep

    10. Heparin may be given intermittently or continuously. With continuous infusions, a bolus (usually 100 units/kg) is given, followed by an infusion of 20,000–30,000 units/day. Some physicians routinely give antacids to patients on anticoagulants.

11. Laboratory: See "Pulmonary Embolism"

    11. See "Pulmonary Embolism."

12. Special: See "Pulmonary Embolism"

    12. See "Pulmonary Embolism."

UNSTABLE ANGINA

1. Admit to CCU

   1. Patients with unstable angina are usually admitted to

the CCU, medical ICU, or medicine floor with cardiac telemetry ("cardiac step-down unit").

2. Diagnosis:
   Unstable angina

2. Unstable angina refers to a variety of clinical syndromes, including cases of patients with chronic angina whose pattern of angina changes in frequency, severity, provoking factors, or responsiveness to nitroglycerin. In some patients, rest angina may have developed. In others, the pain may be prolonged to the extent that the clinician suspects myocardial infarction. Unstable angina usually reflects a change in myocardial oxygen supply resulting from increased coronary vasomotor tone or intraluminal thrombus formation.

3. Condition: Serious

3. Routine.

4. Allergy: NKA

4. Routine.

5. Vital Signs: BP, HR, Temp, Resp q 6 h
   Call physician if:
   BP <90, >170 systolic
   HR <50, >100
   Resp >24
   Temp >38.3°C

5. Routine.

6. Activity: Bed rest, with bathroom privileges

6. Limitation of physical exertion and emotional stress is advisable in the treatment of unstable angina.

7. Nursing:
   Guaiac stools
   In the event of chest pain, please obtain 12-lead ECG and call physician

7. ECG should be obtained if the patient develops chest pain or an "angina equivalent" such as shortness of breath. The presence of transient ST segment elevation raises the possibility of a vasospastic component (i.e., variant or Prinzmetal's angina).

8. Diet: Low cholesterol, no added salt

8. Routine.

9. IV Orders: D5W TKO

9. Routine.

10. Medications:
    O_2 2L via nasal prongs
    Heparin 5000 units IV bolus × 1, then 1000 units/h IV
    ASA: 325 mg PO q d

10. Given the pathophysiology involving intracoronary thrombus formation underlying the majority of cases of unstable angina, therapeutic anticoag-

Nitroglycerin paste: 1.5 inches to chest wall q 4 h—hold and/or wipe off for systolic blood pressure <95

Atenolol 50 mg PO q d

DOSS 200 mg PO q d

Lorazepam 1 mg PO q 6 h prn anxiety

ulation with heparin is advised by most authorities. Intravenous heparin should be adjusted to maintain the PTT at 1.5–2.0 × control (INR 2.0–3.0). The addition of ASA as an antiplatelet agent is recommended by some authorities.

Nitroglycerin is used to control anginal pain. Sublingual nitroglycerin can be used for acute episodes. Nitropaste is employed to deliver continuous nitroglycerin during the acute management of unstable angina. Beta-blockers and calcium channel blocking agents may also be beneficial. (In this patient, beta-blocker therapy with atenolol, which the patient was receiving as an outpatient, was continued.) Intravenous nitroglycerin should be administered to patients whose pain is not controlled with bed rest, optimal oral medications, and nitroglycerin paste. An initial dose of 10 μg/min is titrated up every 5–10 min to control pain or until the systolic blood pressure is less than 100 mm Hg. Some clinicians prefer monitoring with an indwelling arterial catheter when administering intravenous nitroglycerin.

If patients fail to respond to intravenous nitroglycerin and heparin, then emergent coronary arteriography to evaluate for possible angioplasty or coronary arterial bypass graft surgery, is recommended. The placement of an intraaortic balloon pump may be a useful temporizing measure while awaiting surgery or angioplasty.

11. Laboratory
    Admission: CBC, plts, SMA-12, PT, PTT, CPK with MB isoenzyme, U/A, chest x-ray, ECG, PTT drawn 2 h after start of heparin infusion

11. Because the symptoms of unstable angina may mimic those of myocardial infarction, serial ECGs and cardiac enzyme determinations should be obtained. The PTT

Tomorrow AM: CBC, PTT, CPK with MB isoenzyme, ECG

should be followed carefully and the heparin dose adjusted accordingly.

12. Special: Cardiology consultation

12. A cardiologist should be consulted in the treatment of most cases of unstable angina, especially if the potential for cardiac catheterization exists.

DERMATOLOGIC DISEASES

DECUBITUS ULCERS

1. Admit to 4 North

   1. Most patients are admitted to a general medicine floor.

2. Diagnosis: Decubitus ulcer, left heel; peripheral vascular disease

   2. Decubitus ulcers occur at pressure points (heels, sacrum, lateral malleoli, and elbows). They are more likely to occur in patients who have diabetes and peripheral vascular disease, especially those who are bedridden or relatively immobile. Other common cutaneous ulcers are stasis and diabetic foot ulcers.

3. Condition: Satisfactory

   3. Routine.

4. Allergies: NKA

   4. Routine.

5. Vital Signs: BP, Pulse, Temp, Resp t.i.d.
   Call physician if:
   Temp > 38.0° C

   5. Vital signs need not be taken more than once per shift.

6. Activity: As tolerated; no weightbearing on left heel (use crutches or wheelchair)

   6. The most important principle in the treatment of decubitus ulcers is to avoid pressure on the diseased area.

7. Nursing: Position the patient so that no pressure is put on the ulcer
   Decubitus boot for left foot
   Leave ulcer open to the air when not being treated
   Turn the patient q 2 h
   Use an egg-crate mattress pad

   7. Nursing care is of critical importance in the prevention and treatment of decubitus ulcers. Patients need to be carefully positioned and frequently turned to avoid prolonged pressure on any one area. Devices to protect the ulcer area (decubitus boots; sheepskin and egg-crate mattress pads) are helpful. Pressure dressings, such as Ace wrap, and Unna boots are frequently used.
   For stasis ulcers, it is important to request that the foot be elevated at all times. Any ulcer with coexisting edema should be treated with elevation of the affected part. Heat lamps are often used to dry ulcers.

8. Diet: House

   8. Routine.

9. IV Orders: None

   9. Routine.

10. Medications: Débride and clean the ulcer with 3% H_2O_2 t.i.d.

    10. One of the many methods used to treat ulcers is a combination of hydrogen peroxide

Apply Burow's soaks with tepid water to ulcer for 15 min t.i.d. after each H_2O_2 treatment

Routine:

DOSS 250 mg PO every day

Triazolam 0.25 mg PO q hs prn for sleep

MOM 30 ml PO q hs prn for constipation

Codeine sulfate 30 mg PO q 4 h prn for pain

(to débride and clean the ulcer) and wet soaks (to further remove devitalized tissue). The principles are to remove dead tissue, allow granulation to occur, and avoid infection. If infection is present, the patient may require systemic antibiotics. Analgesia is sometimes necessary and may make the patient more comfortable. Topical ointments such as Polysporin or Silvadene can be effective. Also, new "biologic" dressings, such as Vigilon, Opsite, or Duo-DERM, can encourage reepithelialization.

11. Laboratory:

Admission: CBC, electrolytes, BUN, glucose, culture and sensitivity of wound.

11. Blood cultures are indicated if the patient is febrile. Decubitus ulcers should be cultured, even if not grossly infected. Appropriate systemic antibiotic therapy often speeds recovery.

12. Special: None

12. Special orders might include a consultation to develop a plan to prevent recurrence of ulcers or, if the patient were a candidate for reconstructive vascular surgery, a consultation with a vascular surgeon.

PSORIASIS

1. Admit to 8 South

1. Most patients are admitted to a general medicine floor.

2. Diagnosis: Psoriasis

2. Patients with psoriasis are admitted when uncontrollable flare-ups require intensive care that is not easily provided at home, e.g., the modified Goeckerman regimen described under "Nursing." Occasionally, psoriatic patients will be admitted for treatment of secondary infection or severe erythrodermic skin reactions to topical therapy.

3. Condition: Satisfactory

3. "Satisfactory" will be the most common condition.

4. Allergies: NKA

4. Routine.

5. Vital Signs:
   Temp, Pulse, BP, Resp t.i.d.
   Call physician if:
   Temp > 38.0° C
   Pulse > 120

5. Routine.

6. Activity: Ad lib

6. Routine.

7. Nursing:
   Apply 1% crude coal tar ointment in Aquaphor hs
   Each morning, patient is to remove tar with mineral oil, followed by a shower with warm water and soap
   Two hours after the shower, send patient to light box for UV-B light therapy; duration—15 sec less than the measured minimum erythema dose (MED). Patient is to wear eye protectors while in light box
   Apply 0.1% triamcinolone ointment to lesions t.i.d. during the day

7. The so-called modified Goeckerman regimen is performed by the nursing staff. The regimen must be adapted for each patient and is generally prescribed by a dermatologist. Some general guidelines include:

   a. If the patient develops increased inflammation, the potency or duration of the tar and UV light therapy should be decreased, since tar can be quite irritating.

   b. The duration of UV therapy must be determined carefully. Fair-skinned persons will need much lower doses; burning and eye exposure are to be avoided. Subsequent doses are given using the following guidelines: (1) No erythema present—120% of previous dose. (2) Trace erythema present—repeat previous dose. (3) Definite erythema or tenderness present—no UV exposure.

   c. Thick, resistant skin plaques may need treatment with steroid ointments or keratolytics under wet dressings or pajamas. Salicylic acid can also be used.

8. Diet: House

8. Routine.

9. IV Orders: None

9. Intravenous fluids may be required for severe flare-ups.

10. Medications: 1% crude coal tar ointment in Aquaphor
    Mineral oil
    0.1% triamcinolone ointment
    Aquaphor ointment
    Lorazepam 2 mg PO q 6 h; hold for excessive sedation
    Routine: Triazolam 0.25 mg PO q hs prn for sleep

10. In addition to the dermatologic medications that are part of the Goeckerman regimen, some patients may require sedation at bedtime.

    Some dermatologists initially use steroid ointments to treat an acute flare-up, adding tar several days into the treatment. The use of tar should be avoided if erythema is present, since it may worsen the condition. Topical steroids are sufficient to reduce the erythema so that tar may be added to the regimen later.

11. Laboratory:
    Admission: CBC, SMA-12

11. Laboratory evaluation is tailored to each patient. The patient who has been under careful medical follow-up and who is admitted only for psoriasis therapy may require no routine laboratory work. A low serum calcium level, sometimes seen in severe pustular psoriasis, is associated with a poor prognosis. Acute attacks may be precipitated by infection, especially streptococcal infection. The laboratory may be an aid in evaluating this possibility. Other laboratory tests frequently ordered include liver function tests and serum albumin (albumin is lost with scaling skin).

12. Special: None

12. Routine. As indicated.

ENDOCRINE DISEASES

ADRENAL INSUFFICIENCY

1. Admit to Medical ICU

2. Diagnosis: Acute adrenal insufficiency, pneumococcal pneumonia

3. Condition: Critical

4. Allergies: NKA

5. Vital Signs: BP, Pulse, Resp q 1 h × 6, Temp q 3 h × 2, then q 4 h for the first 24 h
   Call physician if:
   Pulse > 120 or < 50
   BP > 160 or < 60 systolic
   Resp > 30 or < 5
   Temp > 40° C or < 34° C

1. Adrenal crisis can be managed on a general medicine floor. Patients with unstable vital signs should be admitted to an intensive care unit.

2. Adrenal crisis is a true medical emergency that often occurs in a patient with preexisting, unrecognized adrenal insufficiency. Infection, trauma, surgery, and prolonged fasting are some of the stressful conditions that can precipitate an adrenal crisis. Rarely, overwhelming sepsis, metastatic carcinoma, or anticoagulation will cause a hemorrhagic infarction leading to acute adrenal insufficiency and crisis.

3. In this example, pneumonia has precipitated adrenal insufficiency. The precipitating stress (often infection) causing the adrenal crisis must be identified and treated. Infection should be strongly suspected when the crisis has developed without an obvious cause.

4. Routine.

5. The patient with adrenal insufficiency will usually stabilize during the first several hours of therapy if glucocorticoid, saline, and water deficits are corrected and the precipitating event is controlled. The frequency of taking vital signs can be adjusted according to the improvement of the patient.

   Blood pressure and respiratory rate are particularly important vital signs in this condition. Hypotension in adrenal crisis usually responds to saline and hydrocortisone, but if circulatory collapse is severe, vasopressors may be required. Hypothermia or hyperthermia may occur and should be treated with routine measures. (Hypothermia should be corrected cautiously and slowly.)

6. Activity: Bed rest

6. Routine.

7. Nursing:
   Daily weights
   I and O
   Encourage coughing and deep breathing
   Incentive spirometry

7. Routine.

8. Diet: NPO for first 24 h, then if nausea is resolved, house diet

8. Routine.

9. IV Orders:
   #1. 1000 ml D5NS with 100 mg hydrocortisone at 250 ml/h
   #2. 1000 ml D5NS with 100 mg hydrocortisone at 125 ml/h
   #3. 1000 ml D5NS with 50 mg hydrocortisone over 12 h (80 ml/h)

9. Most patients in adrenal crisis will have approximately a 20% deficit in extracellular fluid. The key to therapy is to provide adrenocortical hormones and volume replacement. If the patient is in severe shock, volume replacement will be more rapid and prolonged.

   Water intoxication can be avoided by using isotonic fluids for volume replacement. Hyperkalemia, which is usually present on admission, is typically followed by hypokalemia during the second to the fourth liter of therapy. Therefore, serum potassium levels must be monitored and replacement provided as required.

10. Medications:
    Hydrocortisone 100 mg IV (given)
    Ampicillin 1.5 g IV q 6 h
    Hydrocortisone (per IV orders)
    Routine: No routine medications today
    Tomorrow:
    Cortisone acetate 30 mg IM q 8 h
    Triazolam 0.25 mg PO q hs prn for sleep
    MOM 30 ml q hs prn for constipation

10. Most patients will require no more than 200 mg of hydrocortisone in the first 12 hours of therapy. The first dose can be given as an IV push or in the form of cortisone acetate, 50–100 mg IM, followed by an infusion with IV fluids (as noted under "IV Orders"). Mineralocorticoids are not required and may lead to fluid retention (200 mg of hydrocortisone supplies maximal mineralocorticoid activity).

    Patients will usually respond dramatically to the replacement of adrenocorticoids and fluid volume. After the first day of treatment, patients are usually given lower doses of steroid (cortisone acetate or hydrocortisone hemisuccinate, 25 mg IM q 8 h). Steroid doses are tapered according to the patient's clinical status until daily oral replacement doses of 25–35 mg of cortisone acetate (or its equivalent) are reached. The use of routine medications should be withheld until the patient's condition has stabilized. Acetaminophen is not given routinely since glucocorticoids may relieve fever.

11. Laboratory:
    Admission: CBC, SMA-12, UA, CXR (PA and lateral), ECG, blood cultures (2), urine C and S, sputum Gram stain and culture, serum cortisol (already done), electrolytes, STAT; repeat electrolytes (STAT) in 6 h at midnight.
    Tomorrow: Hct, WBC, electrolytes, BUN, glucose

11. The laboratory examination will often reveal hyponatremia, hyperkalemia, and eosinophilia. Cultures are essential to investigate the possibility of infection. Electrolyte status should be followed carefully, since hypokalemia may be severe enough to cause paralysis if it is unrecognized.

12. Special: None

12. As indicated.

DIABETIC KETOACIDOSIS

1. Admit to 5 North

1. Admission is usually to a general medicine floor, but severe acid-base imbalance may require initial stabilization in an intensive care unit.

2. Diagnosis: Diabetic ketoacidosis, urinary tract infection

2. Diabetic ketoacidosis (DKA) occurs as an initial manifestation of diabetes or in the diabetic patient who fails to adjust insulin dosage during an illness or who discontinues the insulin because of poor compliance or the mistaken fear of hypoglycemia. In this example, DKA has been precipitated by a urinary tract infection. Any patient with unexplained DKA should be carefully evaluated for coexistent infection or unrecognized

3. Condition: Serious

4. Allergies: NKA

5. Vital Signs: Postural BP, Pulse, Resp q 1 h × 6, then q 2 h × 3, then q 4 h, Temp q 4 h
   Tomorrow: q.i.d.
   Call physician if:
   BP < 80 systolic
   Pulse > 140
   Temp > 39° C

6. Activity: Bed rest with commode privileges today, ad lib beginning tomorrow

7. Nursing:
   I and O q 1 h × 6, then q 4 h × 3, then every day
   Dipstick urine, chart glucose and acetone once each shift
   Call physician if urine output is < 15 ml/h
   Check capillary blood glucose (fingerstick) 1, 2, 6, 10 h after admission
   Draw blood for sodium, K^+, Cl, HCO_3^-, and BUN (or creatinine) 4, 8, and 12 h after admission; include serum ketones at the first and second blood draws
   Record glucose, K^+, HCO_3^-, BUN, and ketones on flow chart

acute illness (e.g., myocardial infarction, CVA).

3. Condition may range from satisfactory to critical.

4. Routine.

5. The treatment of DKA is facilitated by the use of a flow chart to note important vital signs, laboratory values, and therapy. The nursing staff can record vital signs, urine output, IV therapy, blood and urine glucose and ketones, serum K^+, HCO_3^-, other pertinent lab values, and insulin therapy on the flow chart.

   Most patients have orthostatic changes in blood pressure, indicating at least a 30% extracellular fluid volume deficit. When orthostatic hypotension disappears, the infusion solution can be changed from NS (0.9% saline) to ½NS (0.45% saline).

   Initially, patients with DKA should be observed frequently until their condition shows improvement. Hourly monitoring of vital signs is usually required for the first 6 hours, depending on the patient's status.

6. Routine.

7. The treatment of DKA is designed to correct volume depletion, hyperosmolarity, hyperglycemia, acidosis, potassium depletion, and any precipitating illness.

   Measurement of vital signs, urine output, and concentrations of glucose, potassium, HCO_3^-, ketones, and BUN allows therapy to be monitored. The timing for drawing blood is based on the fact that the greatest fall in blood glucose occurs during the first hour of therapy; thereafter the average fall is 75–100 mg/dl per hour. In many institutions, the nursing staff draw blood

Daily weights

and maintain flow charts and, in so doing, greatly assist with the management of the patient.

In 4–7 hours, most patients will reach a glucose level (about 250 mg/dl) at which time supplemental infusions with glucose must be given to prevent hypoglycemia. Potassium supplementation is usually started during the first 4 hours of therapy and must be undertaken with caution in patients with significant renal failure or low urine output. Hyperglycemia resolves more rapidly than acidosis. Bicarbonate levels reach target values (15–25 mEq/L) in 10–20 hours; persistent acidosis is not a cause for concern as long as the pH or bicarbonate levels are moving toward the normal range. The ready availability of bedside blood glucose measurement has eliminated the need to frequently measure urine glucose and acetone by dipstick.

8. Diet: NPO for 12 h, then clear liquids as tolerated
   1500-calorie diabetic diet tomorrow

8. Most patients with DKA are nauseated and have no appetite. Gastric dilatation, vomiting, and aspiration of vomitus are life-threatening hazards. Nasogastric intubation may be indicated in patients who have a depressed mental status and gastric distention or vomiting.

9. IV Orders:
   #1. 1000 ml NS at 1000 ml/h
   #2. 1000 ml NS with 20 mEq KPO_4 at 500 ml/h
   #3. 1000 ml NS with 20 mEq KCl at 500 ml/h
   #4. 1000 ml ½NS with 20 mEq KPO_4 at 500 ml/h
   #5. 1000 ml D5–½NS with 20 mEq KCl at 250 ml/h
   When blood glucose ≤ 250 mg, IV fluid orders should be changed to contain D5 with NS or ½NS as written

9. Correction of volume (saline) and water depletion is accomplished by the rapid infusion of IV fluids. Most patients with DKA receive about 4–5 liters of fluid in the first 8 hours of therapy. Correction of volume deficit is most important, and normal saline should be infused initially until hypotension disappears. Once orthostatic hypotension is resolved, 0.45% saline can be substituted for normal saline. Infusion rates are based on the severity of the hypo-

tension. When the replacement is adequate, urine output is usually at least 30 ml/h.

If the patient is severely acidotic (pH ≤ 7.1), bicarbonate may be added to the IV infusion. In general, unless significant lactic acidosis is present (suggested by severe metabolic acidosis in the absence of severe ketonemia or renal failure), bicarbonate should not be used if the pH is greater than 7.1.

Most patients have profound deficits of total body potassium, although potassium concentrations may be elevated. An average deficit approximates 5 mEq/kg of body weight. Nomograms are available to estimate the potassium deficit based on the blood pH and potassium concentration. The serum potassium level should be checked every 2–4 hours during therapy until the acidosis and hyperglycemia are corrected and the potassium level is stable. Since most patients with DKA also have deficits of phosphate, a convenient way to give potassium is in the form of KPO_4 and KCl. It is unclear whether replacement of phosphate deficits makes a difference in outcome, and there have been complications with phosphate therapy. If the patient can tolerate oral feedings, potassium can be administered orally rather than intravenously.

Unless glucose is added to IV fluids when blood glucose is lower than 250–300 mg/dl, serious hypoglycemia may occur. Blood glucose concentration can be maintained between 100 and 300 mg/dl by adjusting the glucose infusion rate between 150 and 250 ml/h.

Dextrose infusions are usually maintained for 12–24 hours. After the DKA is controlled, the patient may be given his usual insulin dose along with regular food intake.

10. Medications:

Regular insulin 15 units IV now

Regular insulin 7 units IM now and q 1 h until blood glucose level < 250 mg/dl; then check with physician for further insulin orders

Ceftriaxone 2 g IV q 24 h until the patient is taking PO fluids, then TMP-SMX: 1 double-strength tablet PO q 12 h

Nursing staff is to notify pharmacy when the patient can be given PO medications

Routine: None now

10. A variety of low-dose insulin therapy regimens have been effective in the treatment of diabetic ketoacidosis. The route of administration probably does not make much difference if the patient's response to therapy is carefully monitored.

Beginning the regimen with a bolus of IV insulin (0.33 units/kg) will, in most cases, quickly establish therapeutic levels and produce a desirable fall in plasma glucose and ketones. Thereafter, low doses of regular insulin (about 7 units/h) IV, IM, or SC are equally effective if combined with adequate fluid and electrolyte replacement and close observation of the patient.

If the ketoacidosis is still not under control (i.e., bicarbonate concentration < 15 mEq/L, pH < 7.3, or plasma acetone positive at a 1:2 dilution) after the plasma glucose level is < 250 mg/dl, regular insulin, 4–12 units q 2 h, should be administered until the ketoacidosis is resolved.

During this phase of therapy, dextrose-containing IV fluids should be administered, and careful monitoring for hypoglycemia, hypokalemia, and changes in vital signs should continue. Most patients with DKA treated in the hospital require 50–65 units of regular insulin by this low-dose insulin regimen.

As soon as the patient is able to eat, long-acting insulin can be given at the patient's regular dose. The results of capillary blood glucose measured by fingerstick should be monitored, and additional short-acting insulin can be administered if excessive hyperglycemia occurs.

11. Laboratory:
Admission: Electrolytes, BUN, glucose, ketones, ABGs, CBC, STAT; CXR (PA and lateral), UA, urine C and S
Capillary blood glucose level by fingerstick by nurse (as noted in nursing orders); blood for glucose, electrolytes, and BUN (SMA-6) 4, 8, and 12 h after admission
Tomorrow: SMA-12, phosphorus

11. These orders duplicate what has been written under "Nursing," since nurses will be taking the blood samples in most cases. Monitoring of the patient's plasma glucose and electrolyte levels prevents the consequences of inadequate therapy, i.e., hypoglycemia, hyperkalemia or hypokalemia, or unrecognized lactic acidosis.

12. Special: None

12. As indicated.

HYPEROSMOLAR NONKETOTIC COMA

1. Admit to ICU

1. Admission is usually to an intensive care unit.

2. Diagnosis: Hyperosmolar nonketotic coma, adult-onset diabetes mellitus

2. Hyperosmolar coma is much less common than ketoacidosis but carries a greater risk of death. Most patients are elderly and have either no history of diabetes or mild diabetes controlled by diet or oral drugs. Usually, hyperosmolar coma is precipitated by some event that causes hyperglycemia, i.e., any acute illness, especially infection, drugs (often thiazides and corticosteroids), or consumption of fluids containing large amounts of sugars.

3. Condition: Critical

3. Hyperosmolar coma is a life-threatening complication of diabetes with a high mortality rate, especially in elderly patients.

4. Allergies: NKA

4. Routine.

5. Vital Signs: Postural BP, Pulse, Resp q 1 h, Temp q 4 h
Call physician if:
BP < 80 systolic
Pulse > 140
Temp > 39° C

5. Patients with hyperosmolar coma have a less predictable course than patients with DKA. Frequent monitoring of vital signs is usually required for at least the first day. Neurologic checks are essential

Neuro check q 1 h

until the patient begins to re-gain normal consciousness.

6. Activity: Bed rest

6. Routine.

7. Nursing:
   I and O q 1 h × 6, then q 2 h
   Dipstick urine once per shift, chart glucose and acetone
   Blood glucose by fingerstick q 1 h between lab draws for first 10 h
   Draw blood for glucose, elec-trolytes, and BUN q 2 h × 3, then q 4 h × 3
   Chart glucose, electrolytes, BUN, insulin given, and I and O on flow chart q 2 h

7. Treatment of hyperosmolar coma is designed to correct volume depletion, hypergly-cemia, potassium depletion, any precipitating illness, and acidosis (usually not an im-portant problem). Establish-ing a well-designed flow chart noting the amount of insulin administered, vital signs, fluid intake and urine output, and values of blood glucose, electrolytes, and BUN will make management of the pa-tient easier. Flow chart en-tries can become less frequent as the patient begins to im-prove.

8. Diet: NPO

8. Routine.

9. IV Orders:
   #1. 1000 ml NS with 10 mEq KCl at 1000 ml/h
   #2–6. 1000 ml NS with 20 mEq KCl at 500 ml/h
   Change to 1000 ml ½NS with 20 mEq KCl if patient is no longer hypotensive (BP > 120 systolic, lying and sit-ting)
   Check with physician about infusion rate after 6 h (3.5 L of IV therapy)

9. IV therapy must be tailored to the patient. Volume depletion is present in all patients with hyperosmolar coma, and shock is life-threatening. If orthostatic signs are present (they usually are), extracellu-lar volume is decreased by at least 30% (4.6 L in a 70-kg patient). Fluid replacement status may be judged by the reversal of hypotension, the reappearance of a jugular ve-nous pulse, and urine output of at least 30 ml/h. When blood pressure becomes nor-mal, isotonic saline may be changed to hypotonic half-normal saline. In addition, as serum osmolality decreases, infusion rates should be de-creased.

   Most patients who have survived hyperosmolar coma have received at least 5 liters of fluid in the first 12 hours. Because these patients are el-derly and can have other ill-nesses, great care must be taken to avoid volume over-load. Periodic assessment is of critical importance, espe-cially with regard to volume status and electrolyte balance. Many patients will benefit from monitoring of central pressures with CVP lines or pulmonary artery (Swan-Ganz) catheters.

Profound deficits of total body potassium are found in most patients even if serum concentrations are initially normal. Patients with a normal potassium concentration (as this patient had) will require 10–15 mEq/h, whereas those with concentrations of less than 2 mEq/L or with ECG abnormalities should be given potassium at a more rapid rate but not exceeding 40 mEq/h. Potassium should be administered cautiously to patients who have severe renal failure or low urine output.

10. Medications:
Regular insulin 10 units IV push
Regular insulin 50 units in 500 ml saline infused at 1 ml/min
When plasma glucose level is < 300 mg/dl, decrease infusion rate to 0.5 ml/min and convert all other IV bottles to D5–½NS as ordered above (nursing staff to notify pharmacy of change)
Routine: None now

10. A simple and effective way of administering insulin for hyperosmolar coma is by low-dose continuous infusion. Progress is assessed by hourly blood glucose measurements and determination of plasma glucose levels every 2–4 hours. This method allows gradual correction of hyperglycemia and avoids abrupt decreases in plasma glucose. The infusion rate must be decreased to 0.5 ml/min when plasma glucose is less than 300 mg/dl, and glucose must be added to the regular IV replacement therapy to prevent hypoglycemia. Adjustment of the glucose and insulin infusions will maintain the plasma glucose level between 100 and 300 mg/dl. Glucose and insulin infusions can usually be stopped on the second day, and patients can be given regular food (if tolerated) and a long-acting insulin.

11. Laboratory:
Admission: CBC, SMA-12, phosphorus, UA, portable

11. Laboratory studies will be used extensively to monitor the patient's initial response

CXR, ECG, ABGs, and urine C and S; glucose, electrolytes, BUN q 2 h × 3, then q 4 h × 3

Tomorrow: Hct, WBC, glucose, electrolytes, BUN

to therapy. Critical measurements are plasma glucose, BUN, and serum sodium and potassium. Osmolarity may be calculated by the following formula:

$$\text{Serum osmolarity} = 2[Na^+ + K^+] + \frac{\text{glucose}}{18} + \frac{BUN}{2.8}$$

Laboratory values should be moving toward normal if the patient is responding to therapy. Laboratory studies can be helpful in identifying any precipitating event leading to hyperosmolar coma.

12. Special: None

12. As indicated.

MYXEDEMA

1. Admit to ICU

1. Patients are admitted to either an intensive care unit or a general medical

2. Diagnosis: Myxedema coma, hypothermia

2. Myxedema coma occurs when stress is added to untreated hypothyroidism, leading to decompensation. The untreated hypothyroidism can occur spontaneously, after surgery or radioactive-iodine therapy, or after thyroid hormone replacement is stopped. Patients with hypothyroidism tolerate stress poorly and are predisposed to myxedema coma after trauma or surgery; acute illness, such as an infection; exposure to cold; and administration of central nervous system depressants.

Most patients who have untreated hypothyroidism but who do not have myxedema coma or severe myxedema are not treated in the hospital. Patients who have myxedema and significant cardiac disease may require in-hospital cardiac monitoring during the initiation of replacement therapy.

3. Condition: Critical

3. True myxedema coma has a mortality rate of up to 50%. Hypothyroidism without coma is a less critical illness and almost always improves with thyroid hormone replacement.

4. Allergies: NKA

4. Routine

5. Vital Signs: BP, Pulse, Resp, Temp q 1 h for first 24 h
Call physician if:
BP < 60 systolic
Pulse < 40 or > 140
Resp < 6
Temp < 33° C
Take Temp with special low-reading thermometer

5. Given the severity of myxedema coma, frequent taking of vital signs is mandatory. All physiologic functions are slowed and mental status is severely depressed; hypothermia is present in almost all patients; bradycardia, hypotension, and respiratory depression with CO_2 retention also occur.

To obtain accurate temperatures in the presence of hypothermia, the thermometer must be shaken down to a low level. Special low-reading thermometers are required to measure temperatures that fall below the range of ordinary thermometers.

6. Activity: Bed rest only

6. Routine.

7. Nursing:
I and O
Daily weights
Continuous ECG monitor
Encourage coughing and deep breathing when awake
Keep patient under double blankets at all times to minimize heat loss

7. The nursing staff will carefully monitor fluid volume and respiratory and cardiac status during treatment. Monitoring is important since thyroid hormone replacement therapy can precipitate ventricular irritability, tachyarrhythmias, and myocardial infarction. Hypothermia is best treated by thyroid hormone replacement and measures to minimize further heat loss (e.g., extra blankets). External rewarming is contraindicated, since it may increase oxygen requirements.

8. Diet: NPO until improvement occurs

8. Routine.

9. IV Orders:
#1. 1000 ml D5NS with 150 mg hydrocortisone to run over 12 h
#2. 1000 ml D5NS with 150

9. Fluid and electrolyte abnormalities commonly seen in myxedema include hyponatremia due to inappropriate ADH secretion, extracellular

mg hydrocortisone to run over 12 h

fluid excess, and hypoglycemia. Patients are typically unable to excrete a water load normally, so hypotonic solutions are to be avoided. If hypoglycemia is present, a concentrated solution with 10–50% dextrose in water is preferable to more dilute solutions that can aggravate hyponatremia. Otherwise, the use of normotonic solutions with restriction of water is important.

10. Medications: L-Thyroxine 0.2 mg IV over 2–4 min, L-thyroxine 0.1 mg IV q 24 h until oral medication can be given

10. The treatment of myxedema is designed to restore thyroid hormone concentrations to normal. L-Thyroxine, 0.5 mg IV, restores normal concentrations so that no further administration is necessary for several days. Improvement in vital signs may occur within several hours after the initiation of therapy. The hazard of administering a large dose of thyroid hormone intravenously is the potential for cardiac irritability and myocardial infarction. Therefore, large doses of L-thyroxine should be given with caution to those patients with true myxedema coma. This patient was treated with a more modest dose originally, followed by daily IV infusions, until oral doses could be given. For patients who are not in imminent danger and for those with resolved myxedema coma who are to be started on oral drug therapy, treatment is usually started at a low dose (0.05 mg L-thyroxine daily) and gradually increased to obtain a clinically euthyroid state and a normal serum thyroxine or TSH concentration. Sudden changes in thyroid hormone level may induce undesirable psychologic or cardiovascular disturbances, especially in elderly patients.

To avoid the potential problems of relative adrenal insufficiency associated with myxedema or pituitary insufficiency, it is extremely important for stress replacement doses of corticosteroids (300 mg hydrocortisone every 24 hours; see "IV Orders") to be administered by continuous intravenous infusion. Pharmacologic doses are usually contraindicated, as they inhibit conversion of T4 to active T3.

11. Laboratory:
    Admission: CBC, SMA-12, UA, portable CXR, ECG
    Special: T4, T3RU, TSH, ABGs
    Repeat glucose, electrolytes, BUN, and ABGs in 6 h
    Tomorrow: Electrolytes, BUN, glucose, ABGs

11. Commonly occurring chemical abnormalities in myxedema coma include hypoglycemia, hyponatremia, and hypoxemia and hypercapnia secondary to respiratory depression. These abnormalities should be evaluated periodically to be certain that the patient is responding to therapy and not developing metabolic complications. Mechanical ventilation is sometimes necessary for severe respiratory depression.

Myxedema coma is diagnosed on a clinical basis, but laboratory studies to confirm the diagnosis should be done *before* instituting therapy. The serum thyroxine level and T3 resin uptake (T3RU) are decreased in myxedema. An elevated concentration of thyroid-stimulating hormone (TSH) confirms the presence of primary hypothyroidism, whereas the absence of elevated TSH levels suggests hypopituitarism as the cause. For patients in whom associated adrenal insufficiency is suspected (Schmidt's syndrome or hypopituitarism), serum cortisol and ACTH levels should be determined. In some cases, ACTH stimulation tests should be administered.

Other abnormalities commonly seen in myxedema include sinus bradycardia and low voltage on ECG and pericardial and pleural effusions on x-ray of the chest.

12. Special: None now

12. As indicated.

THYROTOXICOSIS

1. Admit to 4 North

1. Admission is usually to a general medicine floor.

2. Diagnosis: Thyrotoxicosis, atrial fibrillation

2. Hospitalization for thyrotoxicosis should be reserved for severe cases, such as impending or actual "thyroid storm" or if the thyrotoxicosis is complicated by congestive heart failure, tachyarrhythmias, angina pectoris, or life-threatening illnesses. The management of thyroid storm will be discussed under "Medications" below.

3. Condition: Serious

3. Patients in thyroid storm should be listed as "critical."

4. Allergies: NKA

4. Routine.

5. Vital Signs: BP, Pulse, Resp, Temp q 4 h, ECG monitor checks q 1 h
   Call physician if:
   BP >180 or <90 systolic
   >110 diastolic
   Temp >38.5° C
   ECG rate >150 or <60, >5 VPBs/min or doublets

5. Vital signs should be taken frequently during the first day of therapy and then can be taken less often. It is most important to monitor for signs of cardiac dysfunction, although in thyroid storm, severe hyperpyrexia, signs of central nervous system decompensation, severe nausea, vomiting, and diarrhea can occur, and it is just as important to monitor for them.

6. Activity: Bed rest; chair and bathroom privileges

6. During initial therapy, activity is moderately restricted until the peripheral manifestations of hyperthyroidism are decreased.

7. Nursing:
   ECG monitor checks (see "Vital Signs")

7. Nursing care will depend on each patient's presenting complaints. Nervousness and agitation are common in younger patients. Abundant reassurance by the nurse can be most helpful for such patients.

8. Diet: No added salt

8. Because of the possibility of congestive heart failure, salt intake should be limited.

9. IV Orders: Heparin lock

9. Patients with thyroid storm will commonly have fluid and electrolyte deficits that must be corrected.

10. Medications:
    Propranolol 20 mg PO q.i.d.
    Digoxin 0.75 mg PO now, then 0.25 mg PO every day
    Propylthiouracil 100 mg PO q.i.d.
    Multivitamins 1 tablet PO every day
    Routine:
    Triazolam 0.25 mg PO q hs prn for sleep
    Lorazepam 1–2 mg PO q 6 h prn for anxiety and nervousness

10. Drug therapy of thyrotoxicosis is designed to combat the peripheral effects of circulating thyroid hormone, prevent further release of thyroid hormone, treat other manifestations of thyroid hormone excess symptomatically, and provide supportive therapy. Propranolol, or another beta blocker, is the drug of choice to block the effects of excess thyroid hormone. Depending on the clinical state of the patient, the drug is started at doses of 10–20 mg propranolol q 4–6 h and increased until the symptoms are controlled (up to 120 mg q.i.d. but usually 40–50 mg q.i.d.). A beta blocker like propranolol can abolish or control tachycardia and fibrillation, tremor, nervousness, and excess sweating. With careful monitoring, the drug may be given intravenously for thyroid storm at doses not greater than 1 mg/min. Use of the drug is contraindicated in asthma and low-output CHF but may actually improve high-output congestive heart failure. Propranolol will *not* prevent thyroid storm.
    Digoxin is given to patients with congestive heart failure or atrial fibrillation or both. Atrial fibrillation is often refractory to digitalis until the peripheral manifestations of excess thyroid hormone are adequately controlled or excessive production of thyroid hormone is diminished.
    Propylthiouracil or methimazole is used to prevent the synthesis of thyroid hormone. Generally, action is delayed,

so that except for propyl-thiouracil's inhibition of the conversion of T4 to T3, they probably have little effect in the early treatment of hyperthyroidism.

Sedatives may be important to control the nervousness associated with hyperthyroidism. Vitamin supplements are given because of the increased requirements necessary for hypermetabolism.

In thyroid storm, the treatment includes sodium iodide 1–2 g/24 h (often given as Oragrafin, an iodine-containing contrast agent used for oral cholecystography) to inhibit the release of hormone from the thyroid, in addition to antithyroid medication (propylthiouracil or methimazole) and propranolol. Supportive therapy will include hydrocortisone, 200–600 mg IV per day, fluids, electrolytes, and vasopressor agents to treat hypotension, volume depletion, and electrolyte abnormalities. Hyperpyrexia is best treated by a hypothermia blanket. Salicylate may be used, although there is some concern that it may displace thyroxine from binding proteins and further increase the metabolic rate. Oxygen is usually given. In addition, precipitating factors (infection, most commonly) must be identified and treated.

11. Laboratory:
    Admission: CBC, creatinine, electrolytes, BUN, glucose, CXR (PA and lateral), ECG, UA
    Special: T4, T3RU

11. Both T4 and T3RU levels are increased in thyrotoxicosis. A faster method of diagnosing thyrotoxicosis is to determine if the two-hour uptake of radioiodine is increased. If this is to be done, blood for the T4 and T3RU tests should be drawn before the radioiodine is given. Uptake of radioactive iodine can also be used to calculate I^{131} doses if thyrotoxicosis is to be treated with I^{131} later.

Up to 10–15% of patients with thyrotoxicosis will have normal T4 levels and high levels of triiodothyronine ("T3 thyrotoxicosis"). Not all patients need to be screened initially for this entity, especially when the diagnosis is obvious.

12. Special: None

12. As indicated.

GASTROINTESTINAL DISEASES
CHOLECYSTITIS

1. Admit to 5 North

1. Patients with only local signs of cholecystitis can be treated at home with bed rest and appropriate analgesics prior to diagnostic evaluation. However, patients with signs of systemic toxicity will require in-hospital management with intravenous fluids and antibiotics, usually on a general medicine floor.

2. Diagnosis: Cholecystitis

2. Often the diagnosis is not certain on admission.

3. Condition: Serious

3. Routine.

4. Allergies: NKA

4. Routine.

5. Vital Signs: BP, Pulse, Resp, Temp q 4 h
Call physician if:
BP < 90 systolic
Pulse > 140 or < 60
Temp > 40°C

5. Patients with acute cholecystitis are likely to be febrile and tachycardic, and may be hypotensive because of volume depletion or septic shock or both. Taking vital signs q 4 h helps to monitor any improvement in the hypotension or fever and will detect unexpected deterioration of the patient's condition.

6. Activity: Bed rest, commode privileges; ad lib if afebrile tomorrow

6. Routine.

7. Nursing:
I and O
Daily weights
NG suction (constant, low Gomco)

7. The nursing staff should monitor the I and O and the weight of the patient. They will also be responsible for maintaining the NG suction, which helps to relieve nausea and abdominal pain and which may place the biliary tree "at rest."

8. Diet: NPO

8. Oral intake is prohibited in patients with acute cholecystitis until the acute attack subsides. They are then observed without NG suction, usually for 24 hours. Following 24 hours without symptoms and NG suction, diets are usually advanced gradually from clear liquids to a more normal diet.

9. IV Orders:
   #1. 1000 ml D5NS at 200 ml/h
   #2. 1000 ml D5–1/2NS at 125 ml/h
   #3. 1000 ml D5–1/2NS and 20 mEq KCl at 125 ml/h
   Call for next IV orders

9. IV requirements will depend on the clinical state of the patient. Most patients ill enough to require hospitalization will be volume-depleted and should initially receive normotonic volume replacement. When normal volume is restored, IV therapy will consist of maintenance fluids and the replacement of NG suction contents. Usually, the osmolality of NG suction fluid is approximately half that of extracellular fluid.

10. Medications:
    Cefotetan 2 g IV q 12 h
    Meperidine 100 mg IM and hydroxyzine 25–50 mg IM q 4 h prn for pain

10. Cefotetan or cefoxitin is usually recommended as the antibiotic of choice for cholecystitis. For the severely ill patient, some authorities prefer broader gram-negative, enterococcal, and anaerobic coverage (e.g., ampicillin, plus either metronidazole or clindamycin, plus an aminoglycoside such as gentamicin).

    Most patients will require narcotic analgesics. However, most narcotics cause some degree of spasm of the sphincter of Oddi, although meperidine is believed to cause somewhat less spasm. Sedation is helpful in some patients; usually a benzodiazepine (like lorazepam) is used.

11. Laboratory:
    Admission: CBC, SMA-12, SGOT, amylase, UA, CXR (PA and lateral), KUB (upright), ECG, blood cultures ($\times$ 2)
    Send blood for type and cross-match (2 units)

11. The differential diagnosis of acute cholecystitis includes pancreatitis, myocardial infarction, perforating or penetrating ulcer, right lower-lobe pneumonia, acute right kidney disease, and intestinal obstruction. The laboratory studies listed should provide an efficient diagnostic evaluation. Cultures may be helpful to plan antibiotic therapy.

12. Special:
    Schedule right upper quadrant ultrasound tomorrow; indication: R/O cholelithiasis, obstruction
    Surgical consultation as soon

12. Symptomatic cholelithiasis is basically a surgically treated disease. Of all patients with cholecystitis, 95% will be found to have cholelithiasis. It is important to alleviate the

as possible; indication: acute cholecystitis

symptoms and prepare the patient for surgery. Surgical consultation is of critical importance, because, following initial stabilization, the key question is when to perform the surgery. Most surgeons prefer to stabilize the patient with intravenous fluids and antibiotic therapy initially, followed by a cholecystotomy or cholecystectomy. The choice and timing of these procedures will depend on the consulting surgeon.

CIRRHOSIS

1. Admit to 8 South

1. Admission is usually to a general medicine floor.

2. Diagnosis: Cirrhosis, ascites, probable alcohol abuse

2. Cirrhosis alone does not usually require hospitalization. More commonly, side effects of cirrhosis such as ascites, variceal bleeding, jaundice, and fever will lead to hospitalization. In North America, cirrhosis is usually associated with alcoholism.

3. Condition: Satisfactory

3. A "serious" or "critical" designation may be necessary, depending on associated conditions.

4. Allergies: NKA

4. Routine.

5. Vital Signs: BP, Pulse, Resp, Temp q 6 h
   Call physician if:
   Temp > 38°C
   BP < 90 systolic
   Pulse > 120
   Urine output < 100 ml/shift

5. The frequent taking of vital signs monitors the patient for the development of complications, especially sepsis, intravascular volume depletion, hepatorenal syndrome, and alcohol withdrawal symptoms.

6. Activity: Bed rest with commode privileges

6. Bed rest is traditionally the cornerstone of therapy along with measures to improve hepatic function. The use of a commode assures adequate measurement of urine output.

7. Nursing:
   Guaiac stools
   I and O
   Daily weights

7. It is essential to detect any evidence of alcohol withdrawal signs so that early treatment may be instituted.

Observe for signs of confusion, tremulousness, tachycardia, seizures (alcohol withdrawal signs including DTs), and notify physician if withdrawal signs occur 1500 ml total fluid restriction

8. Diet: Minimum 100 g protein, 2500 calories; 500 mg sodium restriction; 1500 ml total fluid restriction (1200 ml diet, 300 ml nursing)

8. In the absence of signs of hepatic coma, a high-protein, high-calorie diet with sodium restriction is indicated, since impaired nutrition is almost inevitably present in Laënnec's cirrhosis. Anorexia is common, and special dietary supplements may be required. Although mild ascites and edema may disappear with bed rest alone, sodium restriction is required in most cases. Fluid restriction anticipates the potential complication of hyponatremia.

9. IV Orders: None

9. Routine.

10. Medications:
Multivitamins 1 tablet PO every day
DOSS 250 mg PO every day
MOM 30 ml PO q hs prn for constipation
No sedatives unless signs of withdrawal appear

10. Multiple vitamins, including folic acid, are important, given the poor nutritional state of most cirrhotics.

Most patients with ascites will require diuretics (spironolactone and furosemide or thiazide), but since these drugs may have side effects, a trial period of bed rest, good nutrition, and sodium restriction is recommended as initial therapy.

Sedatives should not be given routinely to cirrhotics, because they may precipitate hepatic encephalopathy. In general, special care must be taken when prescribing medication for patients with hepatic dysfunction. If sedatives do become necessary, oral oxazepam is a good choice owing to its normal elimination in patients with liver disease. Even so, oxazepam can precipitate hepatic coma and must be used with caution.

11. Laboratory:
Admission: CBC, platelets, PT, SMA-12, SGOT, UA,

11. Diagnostic studies for evidence of dietary insufficiency (anemia, thrombocytopenia)

CXR, (PA and lateral), KUB, ECG
Repeat BUN, electrolytes, glucose in 2 days

or hepatic insufficiency (hypoprothrombinemia, hypoalbuminemia) should be included in most routine laboratory orders. Monitoring of serum sodium, potassium, BUN, and creatinine concentration is critical in patients on diuretics.

12. Special: Diagnostic paracentesis tomorrow—please have paracentesis tray at bedside at 9:30 AM
Patient is to void before study

12. Even in the most typical case of ascites, ascitic fluid should be examined for appearance, cell count, and protein content. A culture should be obtained for any significant clinical change because bacterial peritonitis in cirrhotics may present with only subtle changes. Cytologic examination may be indicated at initial presentation.

DIVERTICULITIS

1. Admit to 5 North

1. Admission is usually to a general medicine floor.

2. Diagnosis: Diverticulitis

2. Not all patients with diverticulitis will require hospitalization. A useful criterion is to hospitalize patients who are ill enough to require intravenous antibiotics and those who must receive nothing by mouth and require intravenous fluids.

3. Condition: Satisfactory

3. The condition varies from satisfactory to critical (i.e., those patients with obstruction, sepsis, and shock).

4. Allergies: NKA

4. Routine.

5. Vital Signs: BP, Pulse, Resp, Temp q.i.d.
Call physician if:
BP < 90 systolic or > 180 systolic
Pulse > 130
Temp > 40°C

5. In more seriously ill patients, vital signs should be taken more frequently. Worrisome vital sign readings are those associated with progressive, uncontrolled sepsis, indicated by persistent fever or shock.

6. Activity: Chair, bathroom privileges as tolerated

6. Depends on the condition of the patient.

7. Nursing:
Daily weights

7. Patients with diverticulitis may develop hematuria from

I and O
Dipstick urine for blood
Guaiac all stools

8. Diet: Clear liquids for now,
   NPO if patient develops
   nausea and vomiting

fistulae extending into the
bladder.

8. The diet order will depend on
   the complications of the diverticulitis. Patients with fever
   and LLQ pain may tolerate a
   liquid diet if there are no
   signs of obstruction or abscess. Those with evidence of
   colonic obstruction and abscess should be treated with
   NG suction and ordered NPO.
   The physical examination and
   the patient's symptoms provide guidelines to diet therapy. During asymptomatic
   phases, patients with diverticulosis are usually treated
   with high-residue diets.

9. IV Orders:
   #1. 1000 ml D5–1/4NS over
   12 h
   #2. 1000 ml D5–1/4NS over
   12 h

9. IV fluids are used to maintain
   a normal volume status and,
   in this case, the physician can
   anticipate that the patient's
   oral intake will not accomplish this. Patients with obstruction or sepsis or both require more vigorous fluid
   resuscitation.

10. Medications:
    Cefotetan 2 g IV q 12 h
    Routine: Triazolam 0.25 mg
    PO q hs prn for sleep

10. Medical therapy for divertic-
    ulitis must be considered in-
    dividually. Cefotetan is con-
    sidered the drug of choice for
    the moderately ill patient
    with diverticulitis. Some pa-
    tients can be treated orally
    with tetracycline because of
    its broad spectrum for
    aerobes and anaerobes. Other
    patients respond favorably to
    treatment with oral metroni-
    dazole. Those with more se-
    vere signs of sepsis usually
    are treated with antibiotics
    having a broader coverage of
    colonic aerobes and anaerobes
    (e.g., ampicillin, plus either
    metronidazole or clindamy-
    cin, plus gentamicin or tobra-
    mycin). Low doses of meperi-
    dine may be required for
    control of pain. Application of
    warm packs to the abdomen
    may give some relief of pain.

11. Laboratory:
    Admission: CBC, SMA-12, UA, CXR (PA and lateral), KUB (flat and upright), ECG, blood cultures (× 2), urine Gram stain and C and S

11. The differential diagnosis includes carcinoma, inflammatory bowel disease, urinary tract infection, and bowel infarction, among others. However, the major distinction to be made is between carcinoma with infection and diverticulitis.

    Initial laboratory work should include the baseline studies mentioned and cultures to try to isolate an organism. Rigid or flexible sigmoidoscopy is helpful to visually examine the lesion if it is within the reach of the sigmoidoscope. Barium enema should be performed after the inflammation has subsided. However, if the radiologist is forewarned of the diagnosis, the test can be done without excessive risk. Either ultrasound or CT can be employed to detect a diverticular abscess. An intravenous pyelogram may be helpful to detect bladder or ureteral involvement.

12. Special:
    General surgery consultation
    Sigmoidoscopy to be performed tomorrow AM

12. Surgical consultation is mandatory from the early stages of evaluation and treatment to long-term management. Many patients with diverticulitis do not require surgical intervention, but consultation is important. Sigmoidoscopy can rule out a carcinoma distal to the lesion and may reveal areas of narrowing and spasm.

GASTROINTESTINAL BLEEDING

1. Admit to ICU

1. Patients with active bleeding, especially those with hypovolemic shock, should be admitted to an intensive care unit.

2. Diagnosis: Upper GI bleeding

2. Upper GI bleeding refers to bleeding proximal to the ligament of Treitz. It is documented by the observation of

hematemesis or nasogastric return that tests positive for blood.

3. Condition: Critical

3. The condition of the patient is determined by the rate of blood loss, the presence or absence of cardiovascular collapse, and the presence of other complicating illnesses. In the early stages of GI bleeding, before volume replacement has been accomplished and the cause of bleeding has been established, most patients will be considered critical.

4. Allergies: NKA

4. Routine.

5. Vital Signs: BP, Pulse, q 15 min, Resp, Temp q 2 h
   Urine output q 1 h
   CVP q 1 h
   Bedside flow chart noting vital signs (including postural BP if no shock), blood and fluid therapy, and results of diagnostic procedures
   Call physician if:
   BP < 60 systolic
   Pulse < 40 or > 150
   CVP > 15 cm H$_2$O
   Urine output < 15 ml/h

5. Vital signs are monitored to assess the volume status of the patient and to guide volume replacement. The presence of shock (systolic BP of less than 90–100 mm Hg in a previously normotensive patient or a decrease of 20–30 mm Hg in a previously hypertensive patient) or postural hypotension (postural drop of more than 10 mm Hg or postural pulse increase of greater than 20/min) indicates at least a 20–25% decrease in circulating blood volume. Other vital signs indicating inadequate circulating blood volume include a urine output of less than 25–30 ml/h or a CVP of less than 8 cm H$_2$O. The most sensitive early indicator of recurrent severe bleeding will be a drop in CVP associated with increased pulse rate. The vital sign values noted at which the physician is called are arbitrary. Ideally, when there is severe GI bleeding, the physician should be constantly aware of the patient's status.

6. Activity: Bed rest

6. Routine.

7. Nursing:
   I and O
   Maintain a bedside flow chart to record vital signs, blood

7. A flow chart allows the nurse to monitor trends and progress easily. Many hospitals have preprinted flow charts to

and fluid input and output, Hct, and the results of diagnostic procedures

Perform gastric lavage with 2 L saline now, then connect to intermittent low suction; repeat hourly and record results; discontinue when there is no evidence of continued bleeding

Foley catheter

monitor GI bleeding. Gastric lavage is used to remove blood clots. This can be accomplished by the nursing staff, but the physician must be aware of the results, particularly of continued bleeding. Lavage also prepares the stomach for diagnostic endoscopy or upper GI x-rays. The procedure can be accomplished with a large-bore NG tube (e.g., #22 Salem sump tube with multiple ports) or an Ewald tube. If nauseated, the patient may be more comfortable with the NG tube left in place.

8. Diet: NPO

8. Routine.

9. IV Orders:
The patient has a right-side CVP and a #16 angiocath in the left forearm
For CVP line: #1 and #2, 1000 ml NS over 1 h; repeat × 1, then call physician for the rate of infusion
For angiocath: Whole blood, 2 units, to run in as fast as possible, then packed red cells, 2 units, over the next hour; check with physician for next blood order

9. Patients with severe shock require immediate volume replacement. The rapidity of the blood replacement depends on the severity of the shock on presentation, response to replacement, and presence or absence of continued bleeding.

The replacement of blood loss should begin as soon as possible. Whole blood is often started initially because of the extra time required for the preparation of packed red cells. Additional blood should be available in the blood bank at all times for the patient with active GI bleeding.

10. Medications:
Lorazepam 1 mg IV now
No others for now

10. Sedation may be helpful, as patients with GI bleeding are usually agitated. In general, the institution of specific therapy (H_2-blocker, antacids) should await a more precise diagnosis, as well as the stabilization of the patient.

For patients with acute GI bleeding caused by ulcer diseases and gastritis, intravenous H_2-blocker therapy is used with or without oral antacids; whereas these agents are unlikely to be helpful in patients bleeding from varices, and more specific therapy is available.

11. Laboratory:
    Admission: CBC, platelets,
    PT, PTT, STAT; SMA-12,
    portable CXR, ECG, UA,
    AST (SGOT), ALT (SGPT),
    pH of NG aspirate
    Repeat Hct q 2 h × 6
    Repeat platelets, PT in 6 h

11. Initial laboratory studies
    should include an evaluation
    of coagulation parameters
    and liver function and enzyme
    tests. The hematocrit is fol-
    lowed at intervals to assess
    the success of therapy. It
    should be remembered, how-
    ever, that the hematocrit is a
    relatively insensitive indica-
    tor of acute blood loss, since
    fluid shifts prevent complete
    hemodilution from occurring.
    In general, in young patients,
    the hematocrit should be
    maintained at 30–35% and, in
    the elderly, at higher levels
    during acute GI bleeding. A
    unit of whole blood should
    raise the hematocrit 3–4%.

    The coagulation parameters
    should be rechecked periodi-
    cally, since patients can de-
    velop platelet and factor defi-
    ciencies with bleeding and
    replacement therapy. If the
    patient is stable enough to
    travel to the X-ray Depart-
    ment, a KUB x-ray should be
    ordered to check the place-
    ment of the NG tube.

12. Special:
    General surgery consultation,
    STAT
    Endoscopy scheduled for 11
    AM

12. A surgical consultation
    should be obtained immedi-
    ately in all cases of GI bleed-
    ing. Surgical and medical
    physicians together should
    decide the need for and tim-
    ing of surgery.

    Endoscopy with or without
    upper gastrointestinal x-rays
    is used in most cases to define
    the cause of bleeding. Ideally,
    the endoscopy is performed
    while the patient is bleeding
    but has been stabilized he-
    modynamically. Subsequent
    management will depend
    largely on the cause of the
    bleeding and whether the sta-
    bilization occurs with initial
    therapy.

HEPATIC COMA

1. Admit to 5 South

1. Patients are usually admitted
   to a general medicine floor or

to the ICU, depending on severity of coma and complications.

2. Diagnosis: Hepatic coma (portal-systemic encephalopathy), cirrhosis

2. Hepatic coma, or portal-systemic encephalopathy, is a state of altered cerebral metabolism produced by the accumulation of various products originating from protein breakdown in the gut. The condition may be precipitated by azotemia, sedatives, narcotics and tranquilizers, gastrointestinal bleeding, electrolyte disturbances, excessive protein ingestion, constipation, infection, progressive hepatocellular dysfunction, or portacaval shunting. Signs and symptoms range from asterixis with confusion and disorientation to unresponsive coma.

3. Condition: Critical

3. Hepatic coma is a life-threatening illness.

4. Allergies: NKA

4. Routine.

5. Vital Signs: BP, Pulse, Resp, Temp q 4 h
Call physician if:
Temp > 38°C
BP < 90 systolic

5. Abnormal vital signs may indicate complications, especially infection and volume depletion (see "Nursing" and "IV Orders").

6. Activity: Bed rest

6. Routine in severe cases.

7. Nursing:
Turn patient q 2 h
Neuro checks q 2 h × 3, then q 4 h
Daily weights
I and O
Guaiac all stools
Notify physician if the patient does not have a stool at least twice a day

7. Bed sores can be avoided by turning the patient frequently. Neuro checks alert the physician to changes in neurologic status, especially evidence of focal findings. Daily weights and I and O are ordered to monitor the patient's volume status. GI bleeding must be detected early and treated. In addition, regularity of bowel movements is essential to minimize the exposure time of the small intestine and colon to nitrogenous substrates.

8. Diet: No dietary protein for now
Give 2000 calories by tube feedings of 1000 ml 60% glucose and 240 ml Microlipid per day

8. Initially, all protein should be restricted, but caloric intake should be maintained at 2000 calories or greater. This can be accomplished by giving 20% dextrose/glucose (800

cal/L) IV or by tube feedings as described. If clinical improvement occurs after several days of therapy, protein intake can be changed to 20–40 g/day and gradually increased as tolerated. Protein must be added cautiously, usually after the patient is improved and stable for 24 hours.

9. IV Orders: None

9. IV therapy commonly consists of blood products for patients who are bleeding, volume replacement (fluid management is directed toward the maintenance of normovolemia and the detection of complications such as hepatorenal syndrome), and potassium chloride to correct hypokalemic alkalosis. If no IV therapy is needed, an IV is not required and may be a source of infection. Unnecessary urinary catheterization should be avoided for the same reason.

10. Medications:
    Sorbitol 50 ml in 200 ml water PO now
    Cleansing enema × 2 now
    Lactulose 30 ml PO (via tube) q.i.d.
    Ranitidine 6.25 mg/h IV
    Vitamin K 10 mg IM qd × 3 days
    Multivitamins 1 tablet PO every day
    No sedatives

10. If the patient is able to protect the airway, oral lactulose and sorbitol may be administered. Sorbitol is effective orally because of its potent laxative action. An alternative that is equally effective is to use lactulose enemas every 2 hours. Lactulose and neomycin are both effective in the treatment of hepatic encephalopathy (probably by reducing ammonia flux). Vitamin K is given to correct the coagulation abnormalities in hepatic dysfunction (as judged by prolonged PT). In severe hepatocellular dysfunction it may be ineffective. Ranitidine is used to prevent or treat GI bleeding that would worsen encephalopathy. Ranitidine, rather than cimetidine, is preferred because of fewer CNS side effects. Continuous IV infusion is now considered the optimal mode of H_2-blocker administration to severely ill

patients. Alternatively, ranitidine can be administered intermittently on a dosage schedule of 50 mg IV q 8 h.

11. Laboratory:
    Admission: CBC, platelets, PT, UA, SMA-12, AST (SGOT), urine culture, sputum culture and Gram stain, ECG, portable CXR
    Tomorrow: Hct, PT, electrolytes

11. Patients should be evaluated by routine baseline laboratory studies, including CBC (for evidence of blood loss, iron, and folate deficiencies), hepatocellular enzymes, measures of hepatic function (PT, albumin), and cultures and x-rays of common sites of infection (CXR, urine and sputum cultures). Paracentesis should always be performed on patients with ascites, since spontaneous bacterial peritonitis is common and may be asymptomatic except as a sign of hepatic coma.

12. Special: None

12. The special studies to be ordered (paracentesis and GI or surgical consultations) will depend on the clinical situation.

PANCREATITIS

1. Admit to 5 South

1. Severely ill patients may need to be admitted to the ICU, but most go to a general medicine floor.

2. Diagnosis: Acute pancreatitis, probably alcohol-induced

2. Pancreatitis is most often associated with gallbladder disease or excessive alcohol ingestion. In this case, the patient has pancreatitis after a drinking "binge."

3. Condition: Satisfactory

3. The severity of pancreatitis varies from moderate illness with epigastric pain, nausea, and vomiting to life-threatening severe shock with hypovolemia and tetany. This patient has pain, nausea, vomiting, and mild hypovolemia.

4. Allergies: NKA

4. Routine.

5. Vital Signs: BP, Pulse, Resp, Temp q 4 h × 24 h, then q.i.d.

5. Taking vital signs monitors the patient's response to therapy and should alert the phy-

Call physician if:
BP < 90 systolic
Temp > 38.5°C
Resp < 6

sician to increasing shock, sepsis, and respiratory depression from narcotics. Low-grade fever is not uncommon in pancreatitis.

6. Activity: Bed rest with commode privileges

6. Routine.

7. Nursing:
I and O
Daily weights
NG suction (constant, low Gomco)

7. The nursing orders are fairly routine for patients with IVs and NG suction. NG suction removes gastric acid, preventing the release of secretin. It is particularly helpful in severe pancreatitis or when there is evidence of ileus. Most patients experience symptomatic improvement of nausea and vomiting while on NG suction.

8. Diet: NPO

8. A diet order of NPO is routine in all cases to inhibit the release of cholecystokinin, which stimulates the pancreas.

9. IV Orders:
#1. 1000 ml D5NS at 250 ml/h
#2. 1000 ml D5NS at 250 ml/h
#3. 1000 ml D5–1/4NS with 20 mEq KCl at 125 ml/h
#4. 1000 ml D5–1/4NS with 20 mEq KCl at 125 ml/h

9. IV therapy for pancreatitis is designed to correct volume depletion (which is most common) and electrolyte abnormalities. In addition, patients may have hypochloremic alkalosis, hyperglycemia, and hypocalcemia. Calcium gluconate, 10 ml of a 10% solution, can be given IV to correct the neuromuscular irritability and tetany associated with hypocalcemia. After correction of these abnormalities, IV solutions are used to provide maintenance fluids and replace losses, including NG suction output.

10. Medications:
Meperidine 100 mg IM q 3–4 h prn for pain

10. Pancreatitis often causes severe pain, and meperidine is usually required. Otherwise, there are no routinely indicated medications. Ranitidine or cimetidine may be helpful in reducing the output of gastric acid and thus preventing the release of secretin.

11. Laboratory:
Admission: CBC, SMA-12, serum amylase, UA, CXR

11. Determining serum amylase level is the single most important procedure in diagnosing

(PA and lateral), KUB (flat and upright; check NG tube placement), ECG

this disorder; however, the results may be normal in the early phases of the disease. In addition, other disorders also cause elevation of serum amylase level, and, in some cases, amylase isoenzyme determination may be useful. The serum lipase level, which stays elevated longer than serum amylase, is also diagnostically useful in some cases. The laboratory evaluation will also help to anticipate complications (hyperglycemia, hypocalcemia) and to assure the proper placement of the NG tube.

Eventually, an ultrasound study of the biliary system may be needed to determine if the pancreatitis was caused by cholelithiasis. After an acute episode, nonvisualization of the gallbladder on oral cholecystogram is common, so x-ray examination is best performed at a later date, although most visualization is now done with ultrasound imaging.

12. Special: None now

12. Depending on the severity of the illness and the certainty of the diagnosis, surgical consultation may be needed to follow a potential "surgical abdomen."

PEPTIC ULCER DISEASE

1. Admit to 5 North

1. Patients are usually admitted to a general medicine floor.

2. Diagnosis: Duodenal ulcer disease

2. Complications of duodenal ulcer disease include pain, GI bleeding, perforation and peritonitis, penetration with pancreatitis, and outlet obstruction with nausea and vomiting. Admission to the hospital may be required for any of these complications. In this instance, the patient had intractable pain that did not improve with outpatient therapy.

3. Condition: Satisfactory

3. Routine.

4. Allergies: NKA

4. Routine.

5. Vital Signs: Postural BP, Pulse, Resp, Temp q.i.d.
Call physician if:
BP < 100 systolic or if there is a postural BP drop > 20 mm Hg
Pulse > 120

5. Taking vital signs monitors the patient for evidence of volume depletion from blood loss or of peritonitis from perforation.

6. Activity: Ad lib

6. Routine.

7. Nursing:
Guaiac all stools

7. Routine.

8. Diet: House diet with no caffeine or alcohol-containing beverages; encourage patient to avoid foods known to exacerbate symptoms

8. The use of special diets for ulcer patients has fallen out of favor. Controlled studies have failed to document their effectiveness, and they may cause complications. In general, most patients are counseled to abstain from alcohol, caffeine, xanthine-containing beverages, tobacco, and salicylates. In addition, foods that make the patient's symptoms worse are to be avoided.

9. IV Orders: None

9. If the patient is not volume-depleted, IVs are not necessary. Patients with other complications will usually require intravenous therapy with crystalloids and blood products.

10. Medications:
Ranitidine 6.25 mg/h IV
Routine: DOSS 250 mg PO qd
MOM 30 ml PO q hs prn if no BM that day
Triazolam 0.25 mg PO q hs prn sleep, may repeat once
Codeine sulfate 30 mg PO q 4 h prn for pain

10. Therapy for a duodenal ulcer is designed to relieve pain and promote healing. This goal is achieved by inhibition of gastric acid secretion by administration of an H_2-receptor antagonist. Continuous IV infusion of an H_2-receptor antagonist is now considered optimal for treatment of severe peptic ulcer disease requiring hospitalization. Upon clinical improvement, therapy can be converted to an oral H_2-receptor antagonist regimen and continued for 6 weeks to allow healing. Omeprazole (40 mg/day) should be reserved for patients with peptic ulcer disease refractory to conventional H_2-receptor antagonist

therapy. Patients with recurrent disease may benefit from therapy directed against *Heliobacter pylori,* if evidence suggests possible infection with *H. pylori.* Currently, therapy is not standardized, but a two-week regimen consisting of colloidal bismuth subcitrate in combination with two antibiotics such as metronidazole, amoxicillin, or tetracycline. If gastrointestinal bleeding is present or suspected, then endoscopy should be performed. If active bleeding is present or a vessel is visible at the base of the ulcer, the use of electrocoagulation, heater probe, or laser therapy is indicated. If bleeding persists, surgical intervention is warranted. Surgery should also be considered for ulcers that cause obstruction or perforation or fail to respond to 6–8 weeks of intensive medical intervention. Other adjuncts of medical therapy of peptic ulcer disease include analgesia (avoiding nonsteroidal antiinflammatory drugs).

11. Laboratory:
    Admission: CBC, SMA-12, serum amylase, UA, CXR (PA and lateral), ECG, Hct
    Tomorrow: Hct; then every other day

11. The laboratory evaluation includes routine baseline studies and tests for complications such as pancreatitis. The possibility of GI bleeding is monitored by periodic hematocrit checks. Other studies used for diagnostic evaluation include upper GI series and endoscopy (in this case, already performed) and determination of gastrin levels to evaluate the possibility of gastrinoma (Zollinger-Ellison syndrome).

12. Special: None

12. Endoscopy would be ordered here, if indicated.

SMALL BOWEL OBSTRUCTION

1. Admit to 5 North

1. Patients with small bowel obstruction (SBO) are generally

followed on a medical service initially. An ICU admission is needed for patients who are in shock from severe volume depletion due to "third spacing." Patients with small bowel obstruction should always be followed closely in the hospital because of the possibility of serious complications such as perforation.

2. Diagnosis: SBO

2. A presumptive diagnosis is made by clinical and radiographic criteria at the time of admission. Although most cases in North America are caused by adhesions from previous surgery, there are multiple other causes which must be considered in the differential diagnosis, including Crohn's disease, hernia, embolus, gallstones, and indigestible food.

3. Condition: Serious

3. Routine.

4. Allergies: NKA

4. Routine.

5. Vital Signs: Postural BP, Pulse, Temp, and Resp q 4 h
   Call physician if:
   BP < 100, > 180 systolic
   Temp > 38.5°C
   Pulse > 140
   Resp > 25, < 10

5. Patients with small bowel obstruction may initially have rapidly changing intravascular fluid status, and development of hypotension is usual if the obstruction is not treated properly and promptly. Many underlying causes of small bowel obstruction are associated with infection. Fever should be considered a clue to a cause other than just adhesions or to a complication, such as perforation, even though low-grade fever is common in simple obstruction. If the patient is unstable over the first several hours of treatment, transfer to an ICU may be necessary.

6. Activity: Bed rest

6. Bed rest is mandatory, owing to the potential seriousness of the condition.

7. Nursing:
   I and O
   NG suction (constant, low Gomco)
   Guaiac stools × 3

7. Strict I and O and daily weights will be invaluable in monitoring volume status and in maintaining IV needs. In addition, high gastric output

Daily weights

correlates with persistent obstruction. NG suction is essential to decompress the GI tract proximal to the obstruction to prevent perforation, and to promote resumption of gastric motility. It will frequently relieve the patient's abdominal pain and nausea, in particular, pain due to distention of abdominal viscera.

8. Diet: NPO

8. Oral intake is strictly prohibited until the obstruction is unequivocally relieved. An NG tube must remain in place until that time.

9. IV orders:
   #1. 1000 ml D5NS over 1 h
   #2. 1000 ml D5NS over 1 h
   #3. 1000 ml D5NS at 250 ml/h
   #4. 1000 ml D5NS at 200 ml/h
   #5. 1000 ml D5–1/2NS and 20 mEq KCl at 125 ml/h
   Call for further IV orders

9. IV requirements will depend on the volume status of the patient. Most patients will require several liters of fluid infused rapidly because of their decreased PO intake, vomiting, and third spacing of fluid into the abdominal cavity. After initial volume resuscitation, the replacement rate will depend on continued third spacing of fluid, NG output, and the patient's BP and urine output. A CVP line may be necessary if 5 liters fails to resuscitate the patient, and a change from NS to lactated Ringer's solution (LR or RL) will prevent development of an "expansion acidosis."

10. Medications:
    Call physician for severe or unremitting pain
    Triazolam 0.25 mg PO q hs prn sleep
    Prochlorperazine 5 mg IV or IM q 8 h prn nausea

10. It is best to avoid narcotic analgesics and to treat the pain by decompressing the viscera. Occasionally, it may be necessary to use narcotics; a mild sedative and treatment of nausea may also be necessary in some cases.

11. Laboratory:
    Admission: CBC, SMA-12, SGOT (AST), amylase, PT, UA, upright CXR, KUB—two views, type and crossmatch for two units packed RBCs, blood cultures × 2

11. Underlying causes of SBO, in addition to adhesions, include gallstones, inflammatory bowel disease, volvulus, incarcerated hernia, and perforation. Ileus secondary to conditions such as sepsis and pancreatitis can mimic frank SBO. It is essential on initial evaluation to seek intraperitoneal free air on x-ray exam-

ination, since free air indicates perforation, which would necessitate immediate surgery. Evidence of infection would argue for earlier surgical intervention as well as antibiotic coverage.

12. Special: General surgical consult ASAP

12. A general surgeon should see the patient on admission and consult regarding the necessity and timing of surgery; surgery may be needed to treat the obstruction as well as the underlying cause or complications. Sigmoidoscopy, colonoscopy, or radiographic contrast studies may be indicated to delineate the level of obstruction and, at times, may be therapeutic in partial SBO.

ULCERATIVE COLITIS

1. Admit to 4 East

1. The patient is usually admitted to a general medicine floor.

2. Diagnosis: Ulcerative colitis

2. Ulcerative colitis follows a chronic course of remissions and exacerbations. Most exacerbations can be treated medically out of the hospital, but severe attacks are life-threatening and require hospitalization.

3. Condition: Serious

3. Severe attacks may require a "critical" designation.

4. Allergies: NKA

4. Routine.

5. Vital Signs: Postural BP, Pulse, Resp, Temp q 4 h
   Daily weights
   Call physician if:
   BP < 90 systolic
   Pulse > 140
   Temp > 39°C

5. Taking vital signs monitors the patient's volume status and response to therapy, especially temperature, which should return to normal with treatment.

6. Activity: Ad lib in room; commode privileges

6. Routine.

7. Nursing: I and O

7. The nurses can observe the transition from bloody diarrhea to formed, nonbloody stools.

8. Diet: NPO except for sips of water

9. IV Orders:
   #1. 1000 ml D5–1/2NS with 40 mEq KCl and 1 amp Berocca-C vitamins over 6 h
   #2. 1000 ml D5–1/2NS with 40 mEq KCl over 6 h
   #3. 1000 ml D5–1/2NS with 20 mEq KCl over 6 h
   #4. 1000 ml D5–1/2NS with 20 mEq KCl over 6 h

10. Medications:
    Hydrocortisone 100 mg IV q 6 h
    Cefotetan 2 g IV q 12 h
    Retention enema of 100 mg hydrocortisone in 120 ml saline b.i.d.
    Routine: Lorazepam 1 mg IM q hs prn for sleep, may repeat once
    No narcotics or anticholinergics

11. Laboratory:
    Admission: CBC, SMA-12, UA, ECG (done); type and crossmatch for 2 units packed red blood cells, stool for ova and parasites and enteric pathogens, blood cultures ($\times$ 2), urine cultures, CXR (PA and lateral), KUB (flat and upright)
    Tomorrow: Hct, WBC, electrolytes, BUN, and glucose

12. Special: Sigmoidoscopy (done); surgical consultation

8. All patients with severe attacks remain NPO to give the colon complete rest.

9. Most patients who enter the hospital are volume-depleted and require replacement therapy. In the "Truelove regimen," at least 3 liters of fluid are given. Hypokalemia occurs frequently, and up to 200 mEq K^+ daily may be required. Many patients will also benefit from parenteral feeding, although it was not ordered for this patient.

10. The "Truelove regimen" consists of no oral intake, vigorous hydration and electrolyte replacement, parenteral and rectal corticosteroids, and systemic antibiotics (tetracycline was used originally). About 75% of patients will respond with remission within 5 days. Patients whose condition has not improved after 5 days of this intensive regimen usually require emergency surgery. Narcotics and anticholinergics are to be avoided in acute attacks, since they may precipitate toxic megacolon.

11. Anemia and electrolyte disturbances are common and can be severe. Transfusions are often required because of blood loss in diarrhea. Since patients are usually febrile, the possibility of underlying infection should be considered. Most patients should have a sigmoidoscopy as part of their initial evaluation. Barium enema is contraindicated during an acute attack, since it can precipitate toxic megacolon.

12. In ulcerative colitis, sigmoidoscopy shows an erythematous, friable, hyperemic mucosa with an exudate of mucus, pus, and blood. Early surgical consultation with joint follow-up provides the best care for these severely ill patients.

HEMATOLOGIC DISEASES

ANEMIA

1. Admit to CCU

1. Admission to the CCU is indicated in this instance because of the severity of the angina that has complicated the patient's severe anemia.

2. Diagnosis: Megaloblastic anemia, angina pectoris

2. Although anemia is common in hospitalized patients, by itself it leads to hospitalization only when it is severe or associated with other problems. Some complications that may lead to admission include angina, congestive heart failure, postural hypotension, shock, and infection or those of other illnesses associated with anemia.

    Anemia is too nonspecific a diagnosis for proper treatment. Microscopic inspection of the blood film has enabled the physician to classify this patient's anemia as megaloblastic. Additional studies will provide more specific information.

3. Condition: Critical

3. This patient, who has a low level of hemoglobin, has developed angina pectoris and hence is critically ill.

4. Allergies: NKA

4. Routine.

5. Vital Signs: BP, Pulse, Resp q 1 h × 6, Temp q 2 h, then VS q 4 h, postural BP qd; continuous ECG monitor
   Call physician if:
   BP < 80 or > 140 systolic
   Temp > 38° C
   Pulse < 40 or > 140
   PVCs > 5/min or couplets

5. Taking frequent vital signs will monitor the patient for increasing hypotension and for development of fever as a sign of infection or transfusion reaction.

6. Activity: Bed rest with commode privileges

6. Routine.

7. Nursing: Continuous O_2 by nasal prongs, 2 L/min
   Guaiac all stools
   Daily weights
   I and O

7. Routine.

8. Diet: House

8. Routine.

9. IV Orders:
   500 ml NS TKO only; 1 unit

9. Transfusions are useful for patients with acute blood loss

packed RBCs over 3 h
Call physician when transfusion is completed

and hypovolemia, chronic hypoplastic anemia or bone marrow failure (especially when complicated by angina, congestive heart failure, shock, or infection), and bone marrow suppression from chemotherapy. If possible, transfusions should be avoided in patients with hemolytic anemias. In patients who have severe anemia and heart disease, the transfusion should be given slowly and should be carefully monitored. In patients with megaloblastic anemia, especially pernicious anemia, transfusion therapy is particularly risky, as their blood volume is expanded and the risk of congestive heart failure is high. Vitamin therapy alone is frequently sufficient; the response is usually rapid and dramatic. In this patient with angina at rest, careful transfusion is warranted, and the physician requests to be notified when the patient's cardiovascular status can be reevaluated.

10. Medications:
Nitroglycerin 0.4 sublingually prn for chest pain; repeat × 2 if no relief, then call physician
Folate 1 mg PO mg qd
Vitamin B_{12} 1000 µg IM today
Routine: DOSS 250 mg PO qd
Triazolam 0.25 mg PO q hs prn for sleep
MOM 30 ml PO q hs prn for constipation

10. Therapy for anemia should usually be directed toward the identified specific cause. Nonspecific therapy is frequently wasteful and may cause harm. Treating B_{12} deficiency with folate may correct the anemia, but the neurologic disease associated with the deficiency will progress without vitamin B_{12} replacement. However, once appropriate studies are drawn, "shotgun" B_{12} and folate therapy may be appropriate acutely, as it may avoid the need for subsequent transfusions. Chronic therapy can be planned on the basis of diagnostic lab studies.

11. Laboratory:
Admission: CBC with smear (done); SMA-12 battery (sent from ER); Fe/TIBC,

11. The blood smear evaluation is a critical diagnostic procedure. It has classified this patient as having a megaloblas-

folate, B_{12} levels, reticulocyte count; CXR (PA and lateral), ECG, UA; type and crossmatch for 3 units packed RBCs

12. Special: cancel bone marrow examination scheduled for tomorrow at 10:00 AM

tic anemia. The possibility of the patient having concomitant iron deficiency is also being investigated.

12. Bone marrow examination will provide a precise definition of the morphology of the anemia, as well as information about iron stores and the presence or absence of malignant disease. However, review of this patient's blood smear suggests straightforward megaloblastic disease, and the patient will be spared the discomfort of a marrow aspiration unless the B_{12} and folate studies are unrewarding. In such patients, the marrow results are unlikely to be helpful unless the smear or course of illness (e.g., peripheral blasts or failure to respond to B_{12} therapy) suggests another disease process.

SICKLE CELL ANEMIA

1. Admit to 6 North

1. Patients are usually admitted to a general medicine floor.

2. Diagnosis: Sickle cell anemia, painful crisis; acute bronchitis

2. Painful crisis, manifested by abdominal, joint and bone, or chest pain, is the most common reason that patients with sickle cell anemia are admitted to the hospital. Infection, in this instance bronchitis, is a common precipitant of crisis.

3. Condition: Satisfactory

3. Routine.

4. Allergies: NKA

4. Routine.

5. Vital Signs: BP, Pulse, Resp q 8 h; Temp q 4 h
Call physician if:
Temp > 38.5° C
Pulse > 140
BP < 80 systolic

5. Because the determination of vital signs may be quite disturbing to the patient who has excruciating pain, they need not be taken too frequently.

6. Activity: As tolerated

6. Most patients prefer to remain in bed, but there is no reason to restrict activity.

7. Nursing:
   I and O
   Encourage oral fluid intake
   Encourage coughing and deep
   breathing when awake
   Nasal O_2, 2 L/min

7. The nursing staff should help to keep the patient well hydrated and, in this instance, should encourage the patient to expectorate. Oxygen therapy is given to most patients with sickle crisis.

8. Diet: House

8. Routine, unless the patient has superimposed heart failure.

9. IV Orders:
   #1. 1000 ml D5–½NS with 44 mEq $NaHCO_3$ at 250 ml/h
   #2. 1000 ml D5–½NS with 44 mEq $NaHCO_3$ at 250 ml/h
   #3. 1000 ml D5–½NS at 125 ml/h
   #4. 1000 ml D5–½NS at 125 ml/h

9. Volume depletion and acidosis are common findings in painful crisis and should be promptly corrected.

10. Medications:
    Meperidine 100 mg IM q 3 h prn for pain (offer q 4 h)
    TMP-SMX 1 double-strength tablet PO b.i.d.
    Folate 1 mg PO every day
    Pneumococcal vaccine 1 dose prior to discharge
    Routine: DOSS 250 mg PO every day
    MOM 30 ml PO q hs prn for constipation
    Triazolam 0.25 mg PO q hs prn for sleep

10. Analgesics should be given as needed to relieve the extreme pain of sickle crisis, although narcosis should be avoided since hypoventilation and the resulting hypoxia may aggravate sickling. However, analgesia is clearly the major therapeutic objective, and medication for pain should be offered at intervals. Meperidine is frequently combined with hydroxyzine 25 mg, especially if the patient experiences narcotic-associated nausea. The treatment of infection and folate deficiency, both frequently seen in sickle cell patients, is also part of the therapeutic regimen in this case.

11. Laboratory:
    Admission: CBC with smear, differential, platelets (sent from ER); SMA-12 (sent from ER); UA, CXR (PA and lateral—taken in ER)
    Tomorrow: Hct, WBC, reticulocyte count, electrolytes

11. The laboratory evaluation determines if acidosis, aplastic crisis, or infection is present. Aplastic crisis is less common than painful crisis but should be recognized and treated promptly, since it may be fatal. Aplastic crisis may be due to parvovirus B19 infection, which may respond to intravenous immunoglobulin therapy.

12. Special: Respiratory therapy personnel to instruct patient in coughing and deep breathing

12. Removal of excessive secretions may greatly improve oxygenation and speed the recovery of this patient who smokes and who has developed acute bronchitis.

INFECTIOUS DISEASES

ACQUIRED IMMUNODEFICIENCY SYNDROME (AIDS) WITH FEVER/ PNEUMONIA

1. Admit to 3 North

   1. Routine.

2. Diagnosis: AIDS, pneumonia, oral candidiasis

   2. Patients with acquired immunodeficiency syndrome (AIDS) often have pneumonia. *Pneumocystis carinii* (PCP) is the single leading cause of pneumonia in this patient population, but other causes include bacteria (e.g., *Streptococcus pneumoniae, Hemophilus influenzae*), *Mycobacterium tuberculosis,* fungi (e.g., *Cryptococcus neoformans, Histoplasma capsulatum, Coccidioides immitis*), and viruses (e.g., cytomegalovirus). Neoplastic conditions, such as Kaposi's sarcoma and lymphoma, may also cause pulmonary infiltrates resembling pneumonia in patients with AIDS.

   This patient has had several days of shortness of breath, fever, and mouth pain.

3. Condition: Serious

   3. Patients with AIDS can usually be admitted to the ward. If respiratory distress, hemodynamic instability, or obtundation develops, admission to ICU may be necessary.

4. Allergies: NKA

   4. Routine.

5. Vital Signs: BP, Pulse, Temp, Resp q 4 h
   Call physician if:
   BP < 90/50
   Pulse > 120
   Resp > 25
   Temp > 38.5° C

   5. Routine.

6. Activity: Bed rest with bathroom privileges (blood and secretion precautions)

   6. Blood and secretion precautions with bathroom privileges are appropriate for patients with AIDS. A private room is not necessary if the patient is capable of good personal hygiene.

7. Nursing:
   Weight on admission, then q.o.d.
   I and O
   Encourage coughing and deep breathing
   Assist patient with mouth care
   Oxygen at 4 L/min by nasal cannula

7. The nursing staff is asked to encourage the patient to cough and breathe deeply to help prevent atelectasis, and to clear bronchial secretions.

   With oral candidiasis, the tongue and mucous membranes of the mouth can become very painful. The patient should be encouraged to maintain oral hygiene.

8. Diet: General, encourage fluids

8. Dyspneic patients may prefer liquids, and patients with gastrointestinal manifestations of AIDS may need to be NPO. If the patient's respiratory rate and temperature are high, extra fluids by mouth or IV are important to prevent volume depletion.

9. IV Orders:
   #1. 1000 ml D5–¼NS at 125 ml/h
   #2. 1000 ml D5–¼NS at 125 ml/h
   #3. 1000 ml D5–¼NS at 125 ml/h

9. Because of suspected fluid deficits due to fever, high respiratory rate, and poor appetite prior to admission, this patient is given maintenance IV fluids.

10. Medications:
    Trimethoprim-sulfamethoxazole 4 single-strength tabs PO q 6 h (80 mg TMP/400 mg SMX per tab)
    Fluconazole 200 mg PO qd
    Prednisone 40 mg PO b.i.d.
    Routine: DOSS 250 mg qd
    MOM 30 ml PO q hs prn if no stool that day

10. Trimethoprim-sulfamethoxazole (TMP-SMX) or pentamidine is the drug of choice for pneumocystis pneumonia in AIDS. TMP-SMX may be given by slow IV infusion if the patient is unable to take oral medications. Pentamidine is administered IV. Patients with AIDS have a high frequency of adverse reactions to sulfa-trimethoprim drugs used to treat *Pneumocystis carinii* pneumonia. Most reactions consist of rash and/or fever, but more serious side effects such as neutropenia may occur. Pentamidine may cause sterile abscesses at injection sites, hypoglycemia, nephrotoxicity, hepatotoxicity, cytopenias, and other side effects. Corticosteroid treatment is now recommended in addition to antimicrobial therapy in the treatment of moderate to severe PCP ($PaO_2 \leq 70$ mm Hg). One cur-

rently recommended regimen is prednisone, 40 mg PO b.i.d. for 5 days, followed by 40 mg PO qd for 5 days, followed by 20 mg PO qd for 11 days. An equivalent dose of IV methylprednisolone can be used for patients unable to take oral medications. Corticosteroid therapy should be initiated within 24–72 hours of initiation of antimicrobial therapy against PCP.

Oral fluconazole can be used to treat severe thrush. Following improvement, maintenance therapy with oral clotrimazole troches should be started.

11. Laboratory:
    Admission: SMA-12, CBC with diff and platelet count, SGOT (AST), VDRL, UA, blood cultures (2), ABG, urine Gram stain and culture, sputum Gram stain and culture, ECG, CXR—done
    Tomorrow: Creatinine, WBC, SGOT, AM sputum for TB culture and AFB stain

11. Since patients with AIDS may have several coexisting infections, cultures from all sites of suspected infection are done. Rectal, urethral, throat, stool, and CSF cultures may be indicated. Because this patient was previously known to be HIV positive, there is no reason to repeat the HIV serologic test at this time.

12. Special: Induced expectorated sputum for cytologic tests—"R/O *Pneumocystis*"—please arrange with respiratory therapist

12. In some hospitals, an induced expectorated sputum sample is examined by the cytologist for *Pneumocystis* organisms. In other settings, a pulmonary consultant is called in to evaluate the patient for bronchoscopy to obtain bronchial or lung biopsy samples for cytologic or pathologic exam.

AIDS WITH FEVER/WASTING/DIARRHEA

1. Admit to 5 North

1. Patients are usually admitted to a general medicine floor.

2. Diagnosis: AIDS, fever, diarrhea, dehydration

2. There are numerous causes of febrile diarrheal syndromes in AIDS patients, including infection with enteric bacterial pathogens (e.g., *Salmonella* spp., *Shigella* spp., *Campylobacter* spp., and

Clostridium difficile), protozoal infections (e.g., giardiasis, amebiasis, *Isospora belli, Cryptosporidium*, and *Microsporidium*), disseminated infection with *Mycobacterium avium* complex (MAC), cytomegalovirus (CMV) enteritis/colitis, and HIV enteropathy. Extensive work-up will reveal a causative pathogen in approximately 75% of patients. Symptoms can range from mild fever and diarrhea to malabsorption to fulminant dysentery and wasting.

3. Condition: Serious

3. Patients requiring hospitalization will usually exhibit signs of significant dehydration or toxicity.

4. Allergies: NKA

4. This patient did not have a history of drug allergy. However, many AIDS patients will develop allergy to sulfa medications during the course of their disease.

5. Vital Signs: BP, Pulse, Resp, Temp q 6 h

5. Routine.

6. Activity: Ambulatory as tolerated

6. Patients should be encouraged to ambulate if possible. Nursing assistance may be required for safety in the unstable patient.

7. Nursing: Usual precautions
   Daily weights
   I and O

7. Universal precautions should be followed in the care of any patient. However, given the risks of HIV transmission to health care workers, universal precautions should be emphasized.

8. Diet: House, as tolerated

8. Patients should be encouraged to take oral liquids, food, and nutritional supplements as tolerated. In general, milk-based substances should be avoided during conditions inducing villous destruction or atrophy.

9. IV Orders:
   D5NS plus 20 mEq KCl/L 250 ml/h × 2 L, then D5-1/2NS plus 20 mEq KCl/L 100 ml/h

9. Dehydrated patients will require intravenous hydration with isotonic saline. Many patients will require supplementation with KCl to replenish

losses. In some patients, intravenous sodium bicarbonate should be considered to correct bicarbonate deficits induced by diarrhea. Severely malnourished patients may benefit from intravenous parenteral hyperalimentation.

10. Medications:
Zidovudine 200 mg PO t.i.d.
TMP-SMX DS 1 tablet PO b.i.d. 3 days/week
Clotrimazole troche 1 PO q.i.d.
Lomotil 1 tablet PO after each loose bowel movement, not to exceed 5 tablets/day
Acetaminophen 650 mg PO q 6 h prn temp > 38.2°C

10. Antiretroviral therapy with zidovudine and TMP-SMX prophylaxis of *Pneumocystis carinii* should be continued in this patient with advanced AIDS and a CD4 count of 30/mm³. The development of neutropenia may require discontinuation of these medications and institution of alternative therapy (e.g., DDI in place of zidovudine, and inhaled pentamidine or oral dapsone in place of TMP-SMX). Oral thrush is treated with clotrimazole troches. Severe thrush may require treatment with oral fluconazole. Antimotility agents are administered for patient comfort, but should be avoided in cases of bloody diarrhea, significant abdominal distention, or ileus. Other drugs such as verapamil and indomethacin have been employed occasionally to reduce the symptoms of AIDS diarrhea. Unusually severe cases may respond to intravenous administration of octreotide (somatostatin analogue). Specific treatment of the underlying cause of diarrhea depends upon identification of the responsible pathogen (see "Laboratory" below). Ciprofloxacin (500 mg PO b.i.d.) can be used to treat enteric infection with *Salmonella* spp., *Shigella* spp., and *Campylobacter* spp. Shigellosis should always be treated with antimicrobials, but because of the risk of promoting a chronic carrier state, antimicrobial therapy should be reserved for only the severely ill patient with intestinal salmonellosis. Patients with

AIDS are at increased risk for *Salmonella* and *Campylobacter* bacteremia, a condition that should be treated with intravenous antimicrobial therapy. Colitis secondary to *Clostridium difficile* should be treated with either metronidazole (250 mg PO q.i.d.) or vancomycin (125 mg PO q 6 h). Oral metronidazole can be used to treat amebiasis or giardiasis. (Note: A course of iodoquinol should follow therapy with metronidazole for the treatment of amebiasis.) TMP-SMX is the drug of choice for the treatment of *Isospora belli*. Disseminated infection with MAC (generally seen in patients with CD4 lymphocyte counts <50/mm³), usually demonstrated by a positive myobacterial blood culture, should be treated in most circumstances. Although the optimal therapeutic regimen remains controversial, a two to four drug regimen consisting of a combination of clarithromycin, ethambutol, ciprofloxacin, clofazimine, amikacin, and rifampin or rifabutin is often employed. The treatment of *Cryptosporidium, Microsporidium*, and CMV enteritis/colitis is controversial at present.

11. Laboratory:
   Admission: CBC, platelets, SMA-12, UA, bacterial blood cultures × 2, mycobacterial blood culture, stool for enteric pathogen culture and sensitivity, stool for *Clostridium difficile* culture and toxin, stool ova and parasites with AFB stain, CXR
   Tomorrow: CBC, electrolytes, BUN, creatinine

12. Special: Social work consultation

11. The laboratory work-up of diarrhea in AIDS is directed toward the identification of potentially treatable pathogens. The AFB stain of stool will allow detection of *Cryptosporidium*. Consideration should be given to colonoscopy and mucosal biopsies if the initial work-up is negative and symptoms persist. Upper endoscopy may be rewarding in selected patients.

12. Social workers play an important role in the ongoing care of AIDS patients and should be involved early in discharge planning.

AIDS WITH FEVER/ALTERATION IN MENTAL STATUS

1. Admit to 5 South

   1. Patients with complications from AIDS are usually admitted to a general medicine floor.

2. Diagnosis: AIDS, fever, alteration in mental status, multiple CNS lesions

   2. In this patient computerized tomography (CT) of the brain performed with a radiocontrast agent prior to admission revealed multiple ring-enhancing lesions with evidence of significant mass effect—a clinical presentation most consistent with CNS toxoplasmosis. Although *Toxoplasma gondii* is the single leading cause of mass lesions of the CNS in AIDS, there are numerous other etiologic factors, including lymphoma, pyogenic bacterial abscess, cryptococcoma, tuberculoma, and progressive multifocal leukoencephalopathy, among others. The presence of multiple lesions renders a diagnosis of toxoplasmosis more likely, while a solitary lesion increases the likelihood of lymphoma. CT with contrast is commonly employed to evaluate these patients, but magnetic resonance imaging (MRI) is more sensitive and may detect mass lesions not apparent on CT.

      Fever and mental status changes in AIDS may occur in the absence of CNS mass lesions. Cryptococcal infection is the most common form of meningitis seen in the AIDS population. However, the clinician must bear in mind that cryptococcal meningitis in AIDS often occurs with only fever and mild to moderate headache. Mental status changes and signs of meningismus may be absent or subtle.

3. Condition: Serious

   3. In general, patients with infections of the CNS should be

considered seriously ill. The presence of "mass effect" on CT implies significant perilesional inflammation and brain edema.

4. Allergies: Penicillin—hives

4. The type of adverse reaction previously experienced by the patient should be specified on the admitting orders and admission note. An "allergy alert" label should be affixed in a visible location on the front of the patient's chart.

5. Vital Signs: BP, Pulse, Temp, Resp q 4 h
Call physician if:
BP <90/50
Pulse >120
Resp >24
Temp >38.5°C

5. Routine. Some clinicians include a list of "neurologic vital signs" to be assessed in these patients.

6. Activity: Ambulatory as tolerated

6. Routine.

7. Nursing:
I and O
Assistant patient with ambulation if necessary
Universal precautions

7. Neurologic deficits may compromise the ability of these patients to ambulate safely without assistance.

8. Diet: General

8. If an impaired gag reflex is present, then a soft solid diet should be ordered to reduce the risk of aspiration.

9. IV Orders: D5NS with 20 mEq KCl/L at 100 ml/h

9. Because of suspected fluid deficits due to fever and poor appetite prior to admission, this patient is given maintenance IV fluids. Because of the potential for exacerbation of brain edema, hypotonic fluids should be avoided. In addition, CNS infection is a common cause of syndrome of inappropriate antidiuretic hormone (SIADH).

10. Medications:
Sulfadiazine sodium 2 g PO q 6 h
Pyrimethamine 100 mg PO qd
Leucovorin 10 mg PO qd
Dexamethasone 10 mg IV × 1 now, then
Dexamethasone 4 mg PO q 6 h

10. In general, empiric therapy directed against toxoplasmosis is started in AIDS patients with mass lesions of the CNS. Biopsy (stereotaxic vs. open) should be reserved for patients who fail to respond to this empiric treatment regimen. Toxoplasmosis is treated indefinitely with a combina-

Zidovudine 200 mg PO t.i.d.
Fluconazole 200 mg PO qd
Ganciclovir 6 mg/kg IV qd
Acetaminophen 650 mg PO q
    6 h prn Temp >38.2°C

tion of sulfadiazine (6–8 g PO qd in 4 divided doses) and pyrimethamine (75–100 mg PO qd, reduced to 25–50 mg/day after 6 weeks). Discontinuation of therapy leads to inevitable relapse. Leucovorin must be administered concomitantly to limit bone marrow depression. Blood cell counts must be followed periodically. Adequate hydration will reduce the risk of sulfadiazine nephrolithiasis.

Dexamethasone is administered to reduce the inflammatory edema causing parenchymal compression noted on the admission brain CT.

Antiretroviral therapy with zidovudine is continued. If neutropenia develops, then DDI should be substituted for AZT.

Intravenous ganciclovir is maintained for suppression of CMV retinitis in this patient.

Intravenous foscarnet can be substituted for ganciclovir if neutropenia should develop.

Fluconazole is used here to treat severe thrush in this patient. Once improvement is noted, fluconazole can usually be discontinued, and oral clotrimazole troches can be used for maintenance therapy.

11. Laboratory:
    Admission: CBC, platelets, SMA-12, PT, toxoplasmosis serology, bacterial blood cultures × 2, UA, CXR
    Tomorrow: CBC, electrolytes, BUN, creatinine

11. Blood counts (especially the white blood cell count) should be followed closely when one is initiating a treatment regimen with a high risk of bone marow toxicity.

12. Special:
    CT scan of brain with contrast—R/O mass lesion in patient with AIDS (obtained prior to admission)
    Social work consultation

12. Either a CT or MRI scan should be obtained to evaluate neurologic deficits or alterations in mental status in patients with AIDS. CT is usually adequate for this purpose, although MRI is more sensitive and can detect small lesions not visualized with CT. Lumbar puncture should usually not be performed in the evaluation of AIDS pa-

tients until mass lesions of the CNS are excluded by CT or MRI.

BACTERIAL ENDOCARDITIS

1. Admit to 5 North

1. Usually, patients are admitted to a general medicine floor.

2. Diagnosis: Bacterial endocarditis

2. In most cases, the distinction between acute and subacute bacterial endocarditis is not critical from a therapeutic point of view. Subacute endocarditis may be more difficult to diagnose initially, and the patient often requires several days of observation while the physician attempts to isolate an organism. A presumptive diagnosis of acute endocarditis is based on clinical findings and should be considered in all patients with fever and heart murmur, especially if embolic phenomena are present. Acute endocarditis involving the aortic valve frequently requires urgent surgical treatment.

3. Condition: Serious

3. Patients with severe valvular incompetence or hypotension should be considered "critical" and may need to be admitted to an intensive care unit.

4. Allergies: NKA

4. Routine.

5. Vital Signs: BP, Pulse, Resp, Temp q 4 h until afebrile for 24 h, then q 6 h
Call physician if:
  Pulse < 50 or > 120
  BP < 80 systolic
  Resp < 5 or > 30
  Temp > 40° C

5. Effective therapy should cause a fall in the patient's temperature within 3–7 days. Hypotension due to increasing valvular incompetence or heart failure is an alarming development.

6. Activity: Bed rest for 24 h

6. Hypotensive and critically ill patients should be on bed rest until their condition improves.

7. Nursing:
  Daily weights
  I and O

7. I and O can be discontinued after several days if urine output is adequate.

8. Diet: House

8. Patients with endocarditis may prefer a liquid diet until their condition improves. Critically ill patients should be NPO, and salt should be restricted in those with heart failure.

9. IV Orders: 500 ml D5W TKO over 24 h

9. Critically ill patients should receive IV maintenance fluids.

10. Medications:
Penicillin G 2 million units IV q 4 h and gentamicin 100 mg IV q 8 h
Routine: DOSS 250 mg PO qd
Triazolam 0.25 mg PO q hs prn for sleep

10. The choice of antibiotic depends on the suspected organisms. Nafcillin, 2 g IV q 4 h, should be substituted for penicillin if staphylococcus is suspected. The antimicrobial therapy should be adjusted once the sensitivities of the organism and the MIC and MBCs have been determined. The duration of antimicrobial therapy is generally 4–6 weeks; for at least the first 2 weeks, doses should be given parenterally. The usual dosage of gentamicin is 1.0–1.7 mg/kg every 8 h.

11. Laboratory:
Admission: Blood cultures × 3, CBC, ESR, UA, SMA-12, CXR (PA and lateral), ECG
Tomorrow: WBC

11. Blood for cultures may be drawn 5–10 min apart and should be taken from different sites. This should not delay the initiation of therapy. Cultures may be negative or slow-growing in patients who have already received antimicrobial therapy. With fastidious or non-bacterial pathogens, or if patients have received antimicrobial therapy, more blood cultures may be necessary.

After 4 days of antimicrobial therapy, blood cultures should be repeated. In the case of suspected subacute endocarditis, multiple cultures should be done over 1–2 days prior to therapy (assuming the patient can tolerate this period without treatment).

The ECG should be examined for evidence of conduction disturbance. The presence of A-V nodal or bundle-branch block suggests the possibility of a myocardial abscess that may require urgent surgical intervention. The ECG should be followed at regular intervals during the course of treatment.

12. Special: Echocardiography—indications: suspected mitral or tricuspid endocarditis

12. An echocardiogram may reveal vegetations or valvular incompetence.

CELLULITIS

1. Admit to 5 South

1. Patients are usually admitted to a general medicine floor.

2. Diagnosis: Cellulitis, lt. forearm

2. Cellulitis is usually caused by a streptococcal or staphyloccal infection. Although many patients are treated effectively as outpatients, intravenous therapy and hospitalization are often required, especially if the infection involves critical closed-tissue spaces such as the palms (where surgical exploration may be required), or if the infection occurs in compromised hosts.

3. Condition: Satisfactory

3. Routine.

4. Allergies: NKA

4. Routine.

5. Vital Signs: BP, Pulse, Resp, Temp q.i.d.
Call physician if:
BP < 80 systolic
Temp > 39° C
Pulse > 120
Resp > 30

5. Taking the vital signs will monitor a patient's response to therapy (usually defervescence) and detect clinical deterioration

6. Activity: Ad lib as tolerated

6. Routine.

7. Nursing: Make certain the affected arm is elevated at all times, especially at night when sleeping

7. Elevation of the affected area is essential in treating the edema of cellulitis.

8. Diet: House

8. Routine.

9. IV Orders: Heparin lock to be used for administration of IV medications

9. Routine.

10. Medications:
Cefazolin 1 g IV q 8 h
Codeine 30 mg PO q 4 h prn for pain

10. The treatment of cellulitis is usually straightforward. Although most patients will respond to penicillin, a semisyn-

Routine:

DOSS 250 mg PO q AM

Triazolam 0.25 mg PO q hs prn for sleep, may repeat once

MOM 30 ml PO q hs prn for constipation

thetic penicillinase-resistant penicillin (methicillin, nafcillin, or oxacillin) or a first-generation cephalosporin is almost always the treatment of choice because some patients, usually those infected with a penicillinase-producing *Staphylococcus aureus*, will not improve on penicillin alone. Currently, there is no way to know with certainty which patients will respond to penicillin alone. After the cellulitis subsides or defervescence occurs, patients may be treated with oral antibiotics on an outpatient basis.

11. Laboratory:

Admission: CBC (taken in ER); creatinine, ECG, CXR (PA and lateral), UA, blood cultures × 2 (drawn in ER); culture and Gram stain of serous fluid obtained from cellulitis (taken in ER)

11. Identification of a pathogenic organism is occasionally possible from blood or local cultures. This information is helpful in deciding antibiotic therapy. Chest x-ray, urinalysis, and ECG need not be ordered routinely as admission tests in uncomplicated cases.

12. Special: None

12. As indicated.

DISSEMINATED GONOCOCCAL INFECTION

1. Admit to 5 North

1. Patients are usually admitted to a general medicine floor. Some patients can be treated on an outpatient basis.

2. Diagnosis: Disseminated gonococcal infection

2. Disseminated gonococcal infection is characterized by tenosynovitis, arthritis with joint effusion, and skin lesions. Rarely, endocarditis and meningitis occur.

3. Condition: Satisfactory

3. Patients usually respond dramatically to therapy. "Serious" and "critical" designations should be reserved for patients with suspected endocarditis or meningitis.

4. Allergies: NKA

4. Routine.

5. Vital Signs: BP, Pulse, Resp, Temp q 4 h until afebrile for 24 h, then q 6 h

5. Routine.

Call physician if:
  Pulse < 50 or > 120
  BP < 80 systolic
  Resp < 5 or > 30
  Temp > 40°C

6. Activity: Bed rest with bathroom privileges

6. Bed rest is indicated to minimize the trauma to inflamed joints.

7. Nursing: Weigh every other day

7. Recording of I and O is necessary only if the patient is unable to tolerate food.

8. Diet: House

8. Routine.

9. IV Orders: 1000 ml D5W TKO over 48 h

9. If food cannot be tolerated, IV maintenance fluids are necessary.

10. Medications:
    Ceftriaxone 2 g IV q 24 h

10. When a patient's condition improves, cefixime, 400 mg PO q 24 h, can be substituted for ceftriaxone. The duration of antimicrobial therapy is usually 7 days. Rarely, penicillin-allergic patients are also allergic to cephalosporins.

11. Laboratory:
    Admission: CBC, UA, SMA-12, cervical, pharyngeal, and rectal GC culture; joint fluid for culture, Gram stain, cell count, glucose, and protein

11. Culture the urethra in males, and obtain pharyngeal and rectal cultures from male homosexuals and from females. Joint fluid complement is high in Reiter's syndrome, and this information may be useful, since the differential diagnosis can be difficult to determine in males.

12. Special: Notify the hospital epidemiologist

12. It is essential to report the disease so that sexual contacts may be found and treated.

HEPATITIS

1. Admit to 5 North

1. Patients are usually admitted to a general medicine floor.

2. Diagnosis: Hepatitis

2. If the type of hepatitis (A, B, or C) can be identified, it should be indicated on admission.

3. Condition: Satisfactory

3. The most common reasons for admitting patients with hepatitis are severe nausea and

vomiting. These patients are usually in satisfactory or serious condition. Less commonly, the condition may be critical owing to hepatic failure and coma.

4. Allergies: NKA

4. Routine.

5. Vital Signs: Temp, Pulse, BP, Resp q 6 h
   Call physician if Temp > 39° C

5. Routine.

6. Activity: As tolerated

6. There is usually no reason to limit activity.

7. Nursing:
   Daily weights
   I and O
   Enteric, urine, and needle precautions

7. The I and O order may be discontinued once food is tolerated. Universal (enteric, urine, and needle) precautions should be followed in the management of all patients with hepatitis.

8. Diet: NPO except for ice chips

8. Most patients are initially NPO, since the reason for admission is usually nausea and vomiting.

9. IV Orders:
   #1. 1000 ml D5NS with 20 mEq KCl at 125 ml/h
   #2. 1000 ml D5NS with 20 mEq KCl at 125 ml/h
   #3. 1000 ml D5NS at 50 ml/h

9. Maintenance IVs are necessary until food is tolerated. When the patient can tolerate food, a high-carbohydrate, low-protein diet should be ordered.

10. Medications: Avoid if possible

10. Patients with hepatitis often have a decreased ability to metabolize medications. Therefore, medications should be avoided if possible. Sedatives and hypnotics may precipitate hepatic coma and have prolonged duration of action. Thus, they are potentially quite dangerous and should *not* be used routinely. Nausea and vomiting will usually cease once the patient is NPO.

11. Laboratory:

    Admission: CBC, ESR, PT, SMA-12, UA, ALT (SGPT), HB_sAg, anti-HAA (hepatitis A antibody, IgM), stool guaiac

11. A guaiac test of the patient's stool is usually needed only on admission to rule out GI bleeding. The bilirubin level (found in the SMA-12) and the prothrombin time provide some idea of the severity of the insult to the liver.

As indicated, hepatitis A and B studies should be ordered for evaluation of the etiology of acute hepatitis. Hepatitis C is an unusal cause for acute symptomatic hepatitis.

12. Special: None

12. As indicated.

MENINGITIS AND ENCEPHALITIS

1. Admit to 5 North

1. Patients are usually admitted to a general medicine floor, although some with severe meningitis require admission to the ICU.

2. Diagnosis: Meningitis

2. The diagnosis may not be precise on admission. Although a presumptive diagnosis of bacterial or viral meningitis may be made, a definitive diagnosis must await the results of a culture. Meningitis includes symptoms of meningeal irritation. Encephalitis is characterized by focal neurologic findings or changes in mentation.

3. Condition: Serious

3. Meningitis and encephalitis are always considered "serious." Patients in a coma or with severe symptoms should be considered "critical."

4. Allergies: NKA

4. Routine.

5. Vital Signs: Temp, BP, Pulse, Resp q 4 h
   Call physician if:
   Temp > 39° C
   BP < 80 systolic
   Changes in mental status

5. Routine. Changes in mental status or development of shock may lead to a change in diagnosis or therapy.

6. Activity: Bed rest with bathroom privileges

6. Routine.

7. Nursing:
   I and O
   Weigh every other day

7. I and O are recorded if the patient is on maintenance IV fluids. Neurologic checks are ordered in some patients.

8. Diet: House

8. Patients may prefer a liquid diet until their condition improves.

9. IV Orders: 1000 ml D5W TKO over 48 h

9. Critically ill patients should be NPO and receive maintenance IV fluids.

10. Medications:
Ampicillin 2 g IV q 4 h

10. Ampicillin or ceftriaxone (in communities with ampicillin-resistant *Hemophilus influenzae*) is the drug of choice for meningitis resulting from an unknown organism. Ceftriaxone 1 g IV q 12 h plus ampicillin is an appropriate empiric regimen for alcoholics and immunosuppressed patients. Therapy for suspected bacterial meningitis should be initiated as soon as possible. The initial therapy should be guided by the presumptive identification of an organism on Gram stain and should be adjusted according to the culture results. If all cultures are negative for 3 days and the patient's condition has improved, antimicrobials may be discontinued. Sedatives are usually contraindicated in meningitis and encephalitis and certainly should not be used routinely.

11. Laboratory:
Admission: SMA-12, CBC with differential, UA, CXR (PA and lateral), blood cultures × 2; CSF for cell count, glucose, and protein; Gram stain, India ink, and culture for bacteria, fungi, cryptococcal antigen, and AFB
Tomorrow: CBC with diff

11. Check a CSF glucose sample against a simultaneously drawn blood glucose sample. CSF Gram stain and culture are the most important studies. Cryptococcal antigen is important in AIDS patients and in other compromised hosts. Patients who have received antimicrobials prior to admission may have atypical symptoms and laboratory findings.

12. Special: Save tube of serum for possible viral serologic tests

12. A CT scan may be useful in diagnosing suspected encephalitis. Temporal lobe abnormalities may indicate herpes simplex and the possible need for intravenous acyclovir therapy.

OSTEOMYELITIS

1. Admit to 5 South

1. Patients are usually admitted to a general medicine floor.

2. Diagnosis: Vertebral osteomyelitis

2. In adults, hematogenous osteomyelitis most commonly occurs in the vertebral bodies. Contiguously spread osteomyelitis usually involves the extremities, especially the lower extremities.

   Osteomyelitis can occur in patients who develop infection after open fractures, surgical reduction of open fractures, insertion of prostheses or other foreign bodies, or penetrating trauma. This patient developed osteomyelitis secondary to an untreated urinary tract infection with bacteremia. The diagnosis was based on his lumbar back pain, fever, and history of urinary tract infection. In most patients, the onset of the illness is insidious and the course gradually progressive.

3. Condition: Serious

3. Routine.

4. Allergies: NKA

4. Routine.

5. Vital Signs: Temp, BP, Pulse, Resp q 4 h when awake
   Weigh every third day
   Call physician if:
   BP < 80 systolic
   Pulse < 40 or > 120

5. The temperature curve is a useful indicator of the patient's clinical course. Monitoring of the other vital signs will detect complications such as progressive sepsis or shock.

6. Activity: Strict bed rest; provide patient with trapeze

6. Parenteral antibiotics and bed rest are the cornerstones of therapy for vertebral osteomyelitis.

   Orthopedic surgeons often use body casts or other methods of stabilization for patients with vertebral osteomyelitis. However, many authorities believe that external stabilization is indicated only for an unstable cervical spine.

7. Nursing:
   Encourage ROM exercises of upper and lower extremities at least twice each day and evening shift

7. Every effort should be made to maintain mobility and prevent boredom in the patient who will have a prolonged hospitalization with strict bed rest. Anything the nurses can do to assist in these tasks is worthwhile.

8. Diet: House, high-fiber

8. With prolonged bed rest, patients tend to become constipated; prunes and high-fiber foods can be quite beneficial in preventing this.

9. IV Orders:
Heparin lock

9. Routine.

10. Medications:
Nafcillin 2 g IV q 4 h
Gentamicin 80 mg IV q 8 h
Meperidine 75 mg PO q 4 h prn for pain
Routine: DOSS 250 mg PO q AM
Triazolam 0.25 mg PO q hs prn for sleep, may repeat once
MOM 30 ml PO q hs prn for constipation

10. The choice of antibiotics depends on the results of the culture and sensitivity tests. Culture results were not yet available for this patient, who had just received a percutaneous needle biopsy of the affected vertebra. Therefore, the patient was treated for both common gram-negative urinary tract pathogens and *Staphylococcus aureus*, the most common cause of osteomyelitis. The choice of antibiotics should be adjusted after the culture results are available.

11. Laboratory:
Admission: CBC, ESR, SMA-12, CXR (PA and lateral), UA, ECG; AP and lateral Lumbosacral spine x-rays—indication: osteomyelitis; Bone scan—indication: vertebral osteomyelitis; blood cultures × 2, urine culture, needle biopsy of bone for C and S, fungi, and AFB (all of the above cultures done)
Repeat CBC, ESR, and creatinine in three days.

11. Cultures are the most important diagnostic test in the early management of osteomyelitis. X-rays may not show changes for several weeks following infection, whereas technetium bone scans are positive early. Significant laboratory values to monitor during therapy include the erythrocyte sedimentation rate, which should decrease if the patient is responding to antibiotics; the hematocrit level, which should increase; and the creatinine level, if the patient is to receive long-term aminoglycosides.

12. Special: consultation to orthopedic surgeon: Please continue to follow patient after bone biopsy

12. Most patients with osteomyelitis should be managed jointly by orthopedic surgeons and medical physicians. Although most patients with vertebral osteomyelitis will respond to bed rest and antibiotics, a complication such as paravertebral abscess may require surgical drainage. The primary treatment for patients with chronic or post-

traumatic osteomyelitis or osteomyelitis associated with a prosthesis or foreign body is surgery, with antimicrobial therapy as an important adjunct.

PELVIC INFLAMMATORY DISEASE

1. Admit to 5 North

1. Patients are usually admitted to a general medicine or gynecology floor.

2. Diagnosis: Pelvic inflammatory disease

2. Patients with PID are admitted to general medical services for a variety of reasons, including uncertainty of diagnosis, pain, need for IV therapy, and the necessity of keeping infected patients out of the obstetric wards. Most cases of PID are caused by gonococcus, chlamydia, and *Mycoplasma hominis,* and the remainder by a variety of aerobic and anaerobic organisms.

3. Condition: Satisfactory

3. Patients usually respond promptly to therapy. The condition can often be serious or even critical.

4. Allergies: NKA

4. Routine.

5. Vital Signs: Temp, BP, Pulse, Resp q 4 h until afebrile for 24 h, then q 6 h
Call physician if:
Pulse < 50 or > 120
BP < 80 systolic
Resp < 5 or > 30
Temp > 40° C

5. The patient's temperature is the most useful vital sign. Septic shock may occur in these patients.

6. Activity: Bed rest with bathroom privileges

6. Routine.

7. Nursing: Weigh every other day

7. I and O should be recorded if maintenance IVs are required.

8. Diet: House

8. Patients may prefer a clear liquid diet if they are nauseated. Seriously ill patients should be NPO initially, since they may need surgery for abscess drainage.

9. IV Orders: 1000 ml D5W TKO over 48 h

9. Seriously or critically ill patients should receive maintenance IV fluids.

10. Medications:
Cefoxitin 2 g IV q 6 h
Doxycycline 100 mg IV q 12 h
Routine:
DOSS 250 mg PO qd
Triazolam 0.25 mg PO q hs prn for sleep

10. When the patient improves, doxycycline 100 mg PO b.i.d. alone should be substituted for IV antibiotics. The patient should receive a total of at least 10 days of antimicrobial therapy. Alternative regimens include clindamycin 600 mg IV q 6 h plus gentamicin 2 mg/kg IV once, followed by gentamicin 1.5 mg/kg IV q 8 h until improvement, followed by clindamycin 450 mg PO q 6 h to complete 10–14 days' therapy.

11. Laboratory:
Admission: SMA-12, CBC, ESR, UA, cervical culture for GC, chlamydia, blood cultures × 2

11. If a culdocentesis is performed, the aspirate should be cultured anaerobically and aerobically and stained by the Gram method. Consider performing a serum pregnancy test, especially if surgery is contemplated.

12. Special: If the patient is infected with GC or chlamydia, notify the hospital epidemiologist.

12. It is essential to find and treat sexual contacts if indicated.

PYELONEPHRITIS

1. Admit to 7 North

1. Patients are usually admitted to a general medicine floor.

2. Diagnosis: Pyelonephritis

2. Patients with pyelonephritis are most likely to be admitted for IV therapy, especially when nausea and vomiting prevent the use of oral antibiotics.

3. Condition: Satisfactory

3. Occasionally, patients are admitted in serious or critical condition.

4. Allergies: NKA

4. Routine.

5. Vital Signs: Temp, BP, Pulse, Resp q 4 h until afebrile for 24 h, then q 6 h
Call physician if:
Pulse < 50 or > 120
BP < 80 systolic

5. Routine.

Resp < 5 or > 30
Temp > 40° C

6. Activity: Bed rest with bathroom privileges

6. Routine.

7. Nursing: Weigh every other day

7. I and O should be recorded if maintenance IVs are required.

8. Diet: House

8. Patients may prefer a clear liquid diet if they are nauseated. Initially, seriously or critically ill patients should be NPO.

9. IV Orders: 1000 ml D5W TKO over 48 h

9. Seriously or critically ill patients should receive maintenance IV fluids.

10. Medications:
Ampicillin 1 g IV q 6 h
Gentamicin 80 mg IV q 8 h
Routine:
DOSS 250 mg PO qd
Triazolam 0.25 mg PO q hs prn for sleep

10. When the patient improves, trimethoprim-sulfamethoxazole, 1 double-strength tablet PO b.i.d., may be given. Ciprofloxacin, 500 mg PO b.i.d., may be used in sulfa-allergic patients. Oral antibiotics should be continued to complete a 10–14-day course of total antibiotic therapy. The only oral antibiotic agents with documented efficacy in the treatment of clinical pyelonephritis are trimethoprim-sulfamethoxazole and the fluorinated quinolones (e.g., ciprofloxacin). If a patient is compliant, then failure is usually due to complicating factors such as obstruction, abscess, or nephrolithiasis. Therapy should be altered pending the results of culture and sensitivity tests or the patient's clinical course.

11. Laboratory:
Admission: SMA-12, CBC, UA, urine C and S, blood cultures × 2

11. The urine culture and sensitivity test is obviously the most critical laboratory study.

12. Special: None

12. As indicated.

SEPTIC ARTHRITIS

1. Admit to 5 North

1. Patients are usually admitted to a general medicine floor.

2. Diagnosis: Septic arthritis, lt. knee, probable *Staphylococcus aureus*; rheumatoid arthritis

2. Septic arthritis commonly occurs in already diseased joints; in this case, the patient had preexistent rheumatoid arthritis.

3. Condition: Satisfactory

3. Often, septic arthritis may be a manifestation of a more serious underlying disorder, which would, of course, affect the condition of the patient.

4. Allergies: NKA

4. Routine.

5. Vital Signs: Temp, BP, Pulse, Resp q.i.d.
   Call physician if:
   BP < 80 systolic
   Temp > 39° C
   Pulse > 120
   Resp > 30

5. The taking of frequent vital signs is generally not required for patients with septic arthritis, unless the patient is toxic with septic shock or has other signs of septicemia.

6. Activity: Up in chair as tolerated, no weight-bearing; may use commode with assistance

6. The septic joint should be protected while the infection is active and until the inflammation has subsided. Weight-bearing and excessive use of the affected part are prohibited. Most patients will prefer to wear a splint to minimize motion and pain.

7. Nursing:
   Assist the patient with passive ROM exercises of the knee b.i.d.; otherwise, keep knee in resting splint; encourage ROM exercise of other joints

7. Although excessive use of the joint is to be avoided, the joint should be taken through its range of motion every day to minimize the risk of ankylosis.

8. Diet: House (offer high-residue foods and prunes if patient is constipated)

8. Routine.

9. IV Orders: Heparin lock

9. Routine.

10. Medications:
    Nafcillin 2 g IV q 4 h
    Aspirin 975 mg PO q.i.d and hs (as taken by patient at home)
    Indomethacin 50 mg PO q hs with snack
    Routine:
    DOSS 250 mg PO q AM
    Triazolam 0.25 mg PO q hs prn for sleep
    Codeine 60 mg PO q 4 h prn for pain

10. High-dose IV antibiotics are indicated for the treatment of septic arthritis and yield good synovial fluid concentration levels. Intraarticular antibiotics are not indicated.
    Patients with rheumatoid arthritis should be maintained on their current regimen if it is effectively controlling disease activity. Long-acting antiinflammatory agents (such as indo-

MOM 30 ml PO hs prn for constipation

11. Laboratory:
Admission: CBC with differential, SMA-12, CXR (PA and lateral), rt. and lt. knee x-rays (AP and lateral—indication: lt. knee, septic arthritis with RA), ECG, UA, blood cultures × 2, joint fluid for C and S, protein, glucose, cell count, differential and Gram stain (already done)

12. Special:
Ask physical therapist to arrange an exercise program for rheumatoid arthritis and to instruct the patient and nurses in exercises for ROM of lt. knee and for quadriceps strengthening
Please have a setup at bedside tomorrow afternoon for repeat arthrocentesis

methacin) are effective in minimizing morning stiffness if given the night before.

Adequate analgesia is important, since septic arthritis is quite painful. Narcotic analgesics predispose the patient to constipation, so attention to bowel regularity and the prescribing of stool softeners are important aspects of routine care for these patients.

11. X-rays of the affected joint are helpful in revealing signs of osteomyelitis as well as for comparison as the illness evolves. Cultures are obligatory before administering antibiotics. In this case, the diagnosis was made by the identification of characteristic gram-positive cocci found in clumps on a Gram stain of the fluid. The absolute white cell count and differential as well as the glucose level of the joint fluid are helpful indices with which to follow the patient's response to therapy. The white cell count will consist of fewer polymorphonuclear leukocytes, and the glucose level of the joint fluid will increase if the patient is responding to therapy. Since several arthrocenteses are performed in most patients for relief of the pain that occurs with the reaccumulation of joint effusion, fluid for testing is readily obtained and the results available to monitor response to therapy.

12. Inhospital physical therapy is extremely important for patients with any type of inflammatory arthritis. The physical therapist can design a program to minimize loss of function and muscle strength. The therapist can also supervise the gradual increase of activity permitted when the infection is resolved.

As stated previously, joint effusions tend to reaccumulate in patients with septic arthritis, and repeated arthrocenteses are necessary to relieve the symptoms and remove the inflammatory fluid. Periodic measurement of the joint fluid white cell count and glucose level (every 2–3 days) can corroborate the clinical impression (based on the fever curve and joint examination) that the septic arthritis is improved or worse.

If the joint fluid remains culture-positive or the white cell count fails to fall, an orthopedic surgical consultation should be obtained for consideration of arthroscopic (or open) drainage of the affected joint.

SEPTIC SHOCK

1. Admit to ICU

1. Some ICUs have standard order sheets to which these orders can be adapted.

2. Diagnosis: Hypotension, sepsis—"septic shock"

2. In the setting of hemodynamic compromise, therapy must be initiated immediately, even before a specific diagnosis of the cause of sepsis is made.

This patient is a 76-year-old man with a history of diffuse atherosclerotic disease. He was found stuporous in his home by a friend.

3. Condition: Critical

3. Routine.

4. Allergies: NKA

4. Information about allergies and regular medications may need to be obtained from family members, old hospital charts, or private physicians, and the orders updated as this information becomes available.

5. Vital Signs: As deemed necessary, at least q 1 h
Call physician if:
BP < 90/50

5. Hemodynamically unstable patients will require very frequent monitoring of vital signs; continuous blood pres-

Pulse > 120
Resp > 25
Temp > 38.5° C or for any other sudden change in vital signs

6. Activity: Bed rest

7. Nursing:
Weight on admission and daily thereafter
I and O
Foley catheter to closed drainage
NG tube to low intermittent suction
Endotracheal tube care per ICU routine
Arterial line care per ICU routine
Swan-Ganz line care per ICU routine
Guaiac all stools
Guaiac NG aspirate q shift

8. Diet: NPO

9. IV Orders:
#1. 1000 ml NS over 15 min—lt. arm—given in ER
#2. 1000 ml NS over 15 min—rt. arm—given in ER
#3. 1000 ml NS at 250 ml/h via lt. arm
#4. 1000 ml NS TKO over 24 h via rt. arm
Two units whole blood via rt. arm when they arrive, each over 1 h
Check with physician for further IV orders

10. Medications:
Vancomycin 1 g IV q 12 h
Ceftazidime 1.5 g IV q 8 h
Dopamine 10 μg/kg/min IV; titrate to maintain SBP >90

sure monitoring with an arterial line is often used.

6. Routine.

7. Because large fluid shifts are anticipated in a patient with septic shock, accurate weights and I and O measurements are essential. A nasogastric tube is placed if vomiting has occurred or if an intraabdominal source of sepsis is suspected. Because of acidosis and obtundation, most patients with sepsis require intubation and mechanical ventilation.

8. Routine.

9. Patients with hypotension should have two large-bore intravenous lines. Frequently, hemodynamic monitoring with a Swan-Ganz catheter is employed to guide fluid and pressor support. If anemia or coagulopathy is present, appropriate blood products may be given to provide volume replacement.

10. Unless clinical evidence suggests a specific organism, broad-spectrum coverage for *Enterobacteriaceae* and *Staphylococcus aureus* is usually initiated. Some clinicians use a combination regimen consisting of a first-generation cephalosporin (or vancomycin) plus an aminoglycoside for sepsis. In this elderly patient, the likelihood of renal toxicity from the aminoglycoside led to the choice of a third-generation cephalosporin plus vancomycin. Other clinicians use imipe-

nem/cilastatin for initial empiric broad-spectrum coverage in sepsis while awaiting the results of appropriate cultures.

Generally, vigorous crystalloid and colloid volume replacement is begun in patients with sepsis. Once the left atrial filling pressure has reached normal or slightly elevated physiologic levels, inotropic drugs are administered by continuous infusion to maintain the systolic blood pressure at a reasonable level.

Because of the risk of "paradoxical" intracellular acidosis, routine use of $NaHCO_3$ should be avoided.

11. Laboratory:

Admission: SMA-6, creatinine, bilirubin, albumin, ABG, CBC with diff, platelet count, PT, PTT, thrombin time, fibrinogen, fibrin split products, UA—done; AST (SGOT), alk phos, blood cultures (2), urine Gram stain and culture, sputum Gram stain and culture; CXR, KUB, lt. lateral decubitus film of abdomen—portable; ECG

At 1200 today: SMA-6, ABG, Hct, platelet count, PT

Tomorrow AM:

SMA-12, AST (SGOT), ABG, CBC w/diff, platelet count, PT, PTT, thrombin time, fibrinogen, fibrin split products

11. Because of rapid fluid shifts and possibly worsening oxygenation or coagulopathy, blood tests are often drawn every few hours or even more frequently.

12. Special:

Prepare patient for LP

Specimens to be sent:

CSF for protein, glucose, cell count and diff, Gram stain and culture

Consult general surgeon:

"Please evaluate patient with sepsis and abdominal tenderness"—done

Ventilator settings:

FiO_2—0.80, AMV 18, tidal volume 1000 ml

12. A lumbar puncture is done to rule out meningitis or encephalitis as the cause of the obtundation.

Sepsis may be the presenting syndrome for many problems for which the definitive therapy is surgical: ruptured abdominal viscus, cholangitis, intraabdominal abscess, bowel infarction, and others. Personal contact between the primary doctor and the consultant is important so that a timely consultation can be made.

For intubated patients, the orders should specify the inspired O_2 concentration (FiO_2), the ventilator mode (IMV—intermittent mandatory ventilation or AMV—assist mode ventilation, also called A/C—assist-control mode), the ventilatory frequency, and the tidal volume. Here a high frequency (18) was chosen to give a minute ventilation of 18 L because of the patient's acidosis. The ventilator settings are reassessed frequently by the physician and changed as dictated by the ABGs and patient's condition.

TOXIC SHOCK SYNDROME

1. Admit to ICU

1. Routine.

2. Diagnosis: Toxic shock syndrome

2. The criteria for toxic shock syndrome (TSS) are fever, rash, hypotension, involvement of three or more organ systems, and desquamation 1–2 weeks after onset of illness in the absence of an alternative explanation.

   This patient is a 17-year-old woman with onset of fever, rash, and dizziness during her menstrual period.

3. Condition: Critical

3. Most patients with TSS require ICU admission because of hypotension or obtundation.

4. Allergies: NKA

4. Routine.

5. Vital Signs: As deemed necessary
   Call physician if:
   BP < 80/50
   Pulse > 120
   Resp > 25
   Temp > 38.5° C
   Or for any other sudden change in vital signs

5. Because of the hypotension, blood pressure is measured very frequently.

6. Activity: Bed rest

6. Routine.

7. Nursing: Weight on admission and q day
   I and O

7. It is likely that a TSS patient will receive large volumes of intravenous fluids; accurate measurement of I and O and weights is essential. A Foley catheter is often placed to monitor urine output.

8. Diet: NPO

8. If gastrointestinal involvement is present (vomiting or diarrhea), the patient should be NPO. In less severe cases, the patient may be able to eat.

9. IV Orders:
   #1. 1000 ml NS IV over 20 min—lt. arm—given in ER
   #2. 1000 ml NS IV over 20 min—rt. arm—given in ER
   #3. 1000 ml NS IV at 250 ml/h—lt. arm
   Check with physician for next IV order
   #4. 1000 ml NS TKO over 24 h—rt. arm

9. Two large-bore IV catheters should be placed. Rapid intravascular volume replacement should be given until the blood pressure rises to 85 to 90 systolic. If hypotension is refractory to volume administration, or if respiratory compromise develops, a Swan-Ganz catheter may be required to guide volume replacement or pressor support. Until BP stabilization occurs, fluid requirements are difficult to foresee; IV fluid orders should be written for only a few hours at a time.

10. Medications:
    Nafcillin 2 g IV q 6 h

10. A penicillinase-resistant synthetic penicillin such as nafcillin probably does not alter the course of the acute illness but prevents recurrences.

11. Laboratory:
    Admission: SMA-6, creatinine, bilirubin; CBC with diff and platelet count; PT, PTT, thrombin time, fibrinogen, fibrin split products; ABG—done in ER; AST (SGOT), CPK, UA, blood cultures (2), urine Gram stain and culture, ECG, portable CXR
    Tonight 2100 h: SMA-6, creatinine, CBC w/platelet count, PT, ABG
    Tomorrow AM: SMA-12, CBC and platelet count, PT

11. Electrolytes are monitored frequently because of the rapid fluid shifts. Hepatic, muscle, renal or hematologic involvement in TSS may cause lab abnormalities. If the clinical situation is unclear, these abnormal lab results may help to make the diagnosis of TSS.

12. Special:
    Cervical, vaginal, rectal, con-

12. *Staphylococcus aureus* is often cultured from the va-

junctival, and nasopharyngeal cultures and Gram stain—all done in ER

gina or cervix in menstruating women with TSS or from infected wounds or mucous membranes in either men or women. If a patient is obtunded or confused, a lumbar puncture is usually done primarily to rule out meningitis.

TUBERCULOSIS

1. Admit to 5 North

2. Diagnosis: Pulmonary tuberculosis

3. Condition: Satisfactory

4. Allergies: NKA

5. Vital Signs: Temp, Pulse, Resp, BP q 4 h
Call physician if Temp > 39° C

6. Activity: As tolerated, in room

7. Nursing:
Weigh every other day
Respiratory isolation

8. Diet: House

9. IV Orders: None

10. Medications:
INH 300 mg PO qd
Rifampin 600 mg PO qd
Pyrazinamide 1500 mg PO qd
Ethambutol 800 mg PO qd
Routine:
DOSS 250 mg PO qd
Triazolam 0.25 mg PO q hs prn for sleep
MOM 30 ml PO q hs prn for constipation

1. Today, relatively few hospitals have tuberculosis wards.

2. Patients are frequently admitted with suspected tuberculosis.

3. The patient's condition may range from satisfactory to critical.

4. Routine.

5. Vital signs may be taken q 6 h if the patient's condition is stable.

6. Confining the patient to his or her room is indicated initially, especially if coughing or expectorating.

7. Routine.

8. Routine.

9. Critically ill patients should receive maintenance IV fluids.

10. Because of the rising incidence of INH-resistant TB, a 4 drug regimen is now recommended for the initial treatment of TB. Risks for INH-resistant TB include inadequate previous treatment, noncompliance with previous treatment, and acquisition of TB in certain regions of the world such as Southeast Asia or the Philippines. In general, antimicrobial therapy for active TB should always include at least two agents to which the

organism is known to be susceptible. Short-course (i.e., 6-month) chemotherapy for INH-sensitive pulmonary TB was developed to optimize patient compliance and thereby increase the likelihood of therapeutic success. The currently accepted 6-month regimen for uncomplicated pulmonary TB consists of an initial 2 months of daily rifampin (600 mg), INH (300 mg), and pyrazinamide (30 mg/kg), followed by 4 months of daily rifampin and INH. Supplemental pyridoxine (50 mg/day) should be given to patients with suspect dietary habits for the duration of INH therapy. While sensitivity data are being awaited, ethambutol (15 mg/kg/day) should be added to the treatment regimen. Far-advanced pulmonary TB and miliary, meningeal, or pericardial TB should receive 9 to 12-month regimens of triple-drug therapy (INH, rifampin, and ethambutol; INH, rifampin, and streptomycin; or INH, ethambutol, and streptomycin).

11. Laboratory:
    CXR (PA and lateral), CBC, SMA-12, ALT (SGOT), UA, morning sputums for culture and AFB stain × 3, intermediate-strength PPD and simultaneous control skin tests, ECG, HIV serology

11. AFB smears and cultures are the cornerstones of diagnosis. If the patient is not producing adequate sputum for testing, three morning gastric aspirates may be needed. Baseline AST (SGPT), ALT (SGOT), and bilirubin levels should be obtained if the patient is being treated with INH. Because of the increased incidence of TB in the HIV-positive patient population, HIV testing should be considered for patients with newly diagnosed TB.

12. Special: None

12. Audiometry should be performed if the patient is receiving streptomycin. If carcinoma is suspected, consider sending a sputum sample for cytologic testing using bron-

choscopy, if necessary, to obtain an adequate specimen. Other tests that might be informative are LP, bone marrow study, liver biopsy, thoracentesis, and pericardiocentesis. Contact the public health department when a definite diagnosis of TB has been made.

NEOPLASTIC DISEASES

Patients with cancer are admitted to the hospital for diagnosis and staging, chemotherapy, and treatment of the complications resulting from their malignant disease and its therapy. Those with malignant disease present a variety of diagnostic and therapeutic challenges, and approaches to patient care must be highly individualized. The purpose of this section is to provide examples of orders written for situations that occur commonly in patients with cancer, including orders for patients receiving in-hospital chemotherapy and for patients with complications of neoplastic diseases.

COMPLICATIONS OF NEOPLASTIC DISEASES

Fever and Infection

1. Admit to 8 South

1. Patients are usually admitted to a general medicine floor or oncology unit.

2. Diagnosis: Fever, leukopenia, non-Hodgkin's lymphoma, s/p chemotherapy ending 7 days ago

2. Fever and infection are the most common complications that occur in patients with malignant disease. When fever occurs in such patients, it should be assumed that it represents infection until another cause is found. Patients with a fever and fewer than 500 granulocytes/mm^3 should be treated as if they have a bacterial infection (65% of patients with fewer than 500 neutrophils and temperatures of 101°F [38.3°C] or greater have a bacterial infection). Patients should be evaluated for a specific source of infection and physicians should attempt to isolate an organism, but antimicrobial therapy should not be delayed until a definitive diagnosis is made. Therapy should be initiated immediately, since up to 25% of these patients may die in 24 hours if not treated with antibiotics.

3. Condition: Serious

3. The condition may be critical in many instances.

4. Allergies: NKA

4. Routine.

5. Vital Signs: Temp, Pulse, BP, Resp q 4 h
Call physician if:
BP < 90 systolic

5. Routine. Septic shock and respiratory insufficiency are serious complications.

Pulse > 120
Resp > 30
Temp > 39°C

6. Activity: Restrict to room

7. Nursing:
Mask precautions; strict handwashing precautions at all times
No rectal temperatures, exams, or medications
Sitz baths prn for hemorrhoids or rectal irritation
I and O
Mouth care

8. Diet: House; push fluids

9. IV Orders: Heparin lock

10. Medications:
Ceftazidime 1.5 g IV q 8 h
Routine:
Acetaminophen 650 mg PO q 4 h prn for Temp > 38°C
DOSS 250 mg PO qd
MOM 30 ml PO q hs prn for constipation
Triazolam 0.25 mg PO q hs prn for sleep, may repeat once
Nystatin oral suspension 400,000 units, swish and swallow, q.i.d.

6. Routine.

7. Isolation procedures vary at different institutions. However, most clinicians agree that an attempt should be made to protect leukopenic patients from the infections carried by hospital personnel. This is especially important with highly contagious and potentially lethal infections such as varicella-zoster.

Manipulation of the rectal area is a potential cause of bacteremia and should be avoided, although the area should be inspected daily. Rectal disease must be treated promptly, since hemorrhoids and rectal inflammation can quickly lead to abscess formation and sepsis.

8. Routine.

9. Routine.

10. Empiric antibiotic therapy is designed to cover gram-negative organisms (especially *Pseudomonas aeruginosa*) commonly found in febrile leukopenic patients. However, *Staphylococcus epidermidis* infections are becoming more common, especially in patients with Hickman (or other indwelling) catheters. There is no ideal antibiotic regimen. An antipseudomonal third-generation cephalosporin, like ceftazidime in this case, with or without an aminoglycoside or another beta-lactam antibiotic, provides effective initial empiric therapy for most neutropenic patients. Vancomycin may be added to this regimen, especially if an indwelling catheter is present. If blood cultures are positive, then therapy is generally continued for 14 days, with extension until neutro-

penia resolves. If blood cultures are negative, then antibiotics may be discontinued when the granulocyte count is greater than 500 mm^3. Antibiotic therapy can be more specific if a source of infection is identified. If a patient remains febrile after 5–7 days of empiric broad-spectrum antimicrobial therapy, superinfection, particularly with fungi, must be considered. Amphotericin B therapy is often recommended at dosages of 0.5 mg/kg/day, along with antibacterial agents, until the neutropenia resolves.

Proper mouth care is extremely important. Any oral candidiasis should be treated promptly.

Therapy with granulocyte-colony stimulating factor (G-CSF) can be employed to hasten the recovery from neutropenia following cytotoxic chemotherapy.

11. Laboratory:
    Admission: CBC with absolute polys, SMA-12, uric acid, CXR (PA and lateral), UA, blood cultures × 2, urine and sputum cultures, Gram stain of sputum; type and crossmatch 2 units packed RBCs (done)
    Tomorrow: Hct, WBC with absolute polys, platelet count, creatinine, and electrolytes

11. Hematologic parameters (granulocyte and platelet counts) should be evaluated frequently. Laboratory studies to determine the source of the fever usually include chest films and multiple cultures. Transfusions of packed cells and platelets are often required for patients with disease-associated or chemotherapy-induced leukopenia. Repeated examinations and cultures will often reveal a source of fever not obvious on the initial work-up.

12. Special: None

12. As indicated.

Hypercalcemia

1. Admit to 8 South

1. Patients are usually admitted to a general medicine floor.

2. Diagnosis: Hypercalcemia

2. Hypercalcemia as a complication of malignant disease is

most commonly encountered in carcinomas of the breast, lung, prostate, head, and neck and in multiple myeloma. It is a serious illness demanding prompt recognition and therapy. Symptoms include anorexia, nausea, vomiting, abdominal and bone pain, constipation, polyuria, confusion, psychosis, obtundation, and finally coma. The most important therapeutic measure is volume replacement, since almost all patients are volume depleted. Volume expansion itself will cause a calcium diuresis and will lower the serum calcium level to some degree in virtually all patients.

3. Condition: Serious

3. The condition may be critical, never satisfactory.

4. Allergies: NKA

4. Routine.

5. Vital Signs: BP, Pulse, Resp, q 2 h; Temp q 4 h
   Urine output q 1 h
   CVP readings q 1 h
   Call physician if:
      Temp > 38.5°C
      BP < 90 systolic
      Urine output < 300 ml in 4 h
      CVP > 12
      Resp > 30

5. Because of vigorous volume expansion therapy and saline diuresis, assessment of the patient for adequacy of urine output and evidence of volume overload is of critical importance.

6. Activity: Bed rest until calcium level is lowered, then encourage activity

6. Immobilization frequently causes hypercalcemia. Prolonged immobilization should be avoided, and ambulation should be encouraged as soon as patients have recovered from an acute episode.

7. Nursing:
   Strict I and O
   Foley catheter
   Keep flow chart of hourly urine output, BP, electrolytes, CVP, calcium, BUN, creatinine, IV fluids, and furosemide therapy

7. Flow charts are extremely helpful in the management of patients who receive vigorous IV therapy and who require frequent monitoring of electrolyte levels.

8. Diet: NPO until nausea is resolved, then full liquids and low-calcium diet

8. Routine.

9. IV Orders:

#1. 1000 ml NS over 2 h

#2. 1000 ml ½NS with 20 mEq KCl over 2 h

Alternate NS (1000 ml) with ½NS (1000 ml) with 20 mEq KCl at rate of 500 ml/h until CVP > 10; decrease rate to 350 ml/h when CVP > 10

9. Vigorous hydration is the key to the early management of hypercalcemia. In patients without heart disease, rapid volume expansion, as outlined, is indicated. When volume expansion has been achieved, rapid saline infusion is continued, and furosemide therapy is initiated to augment calciuria and prevent fluid volume overload. The goals of treatment are to maintain urine output above 300 ml/h and to replace urinary losses of Na^+ and K^+.

10. Medications:

After CVP ≥ 10, give furosemide 20 mg IV q 2 h prn for urine output of < 300 ml/h

Etidronate 450 mg IV over 2–3 h now

Routine:

Meperidine 75 mg IM or PO q 4 h prn for pain

Prochlorperazine 5 mg IV q 4 h prn for nausea

When not NPO: DOSS 250 mg PO qd

Acetaminophen 650 mg PO q 4 h prn for Temp > 38°C

10. Many patients with hypercalcemia will respond simply to saline and furosemide diuresis. However, patients with malignant disease and a high calcium level will frequently require additional therapy. This patient required additional therapy with etidronate, a bisphosphonate. This drug does not act as quickly as saline and furosemide but it is especially helpful in patients with malignant disease and refractory hypercalcemia. Etidronate should be administered at a dose of 7.5 mg/kg IV qd over 2–3 h for 3–5 days. This acute therapy can be followed with maintenance oral etidronate at a dose of 20 mg/kg/day. Osteomalacia can occur with prolonged use of etidronate. Other agents potentially useful for selected patients with hypercalcemia secondary to malignant disease include calcitonin, mithramycin, and gallium nitrate. Glucocorticoids may be especially useful for hypercalcemia due to multiple myeloma or other malignant hematologic diseases.

11. Laboratory:

Admission: CBC, platelet count, SMA-12, phosphorus, UA, urine C and S, CXR (PA and lateral), ECG; repeat electrolytes, BUN,

11. The electrolyte levels (calcium and urine Na^+ and K^+) should be followed frequently, especially during the first 24 hours. Thrombocytopenia is a complication of mithramycin

and glucose in 6 hours and q 6 h × 3, STAT; urine Na$^+$ and K$^+$ in 6 hours; Ca^{++} in 12 hours, STAT
Tomorrow: CBC, platelet count, Ca^{++}, STAT

use and must be watched for. If hypokalemia is present, KCl requirements will be greater, especially in patients who are receiving corticosteroids.

12. Special: None

12. As indicated.

Malignant Effusion

1. Admit to 8 South

1. Usually, patients are admitted to a general medicine floor.

2. Diagnosis: Breast cancer, metastatic malignant pleural effusion

2. Malignant effusions commonly accumulate in the pleural and peritoneal spaces. They are associated with tumor extension or implants, free malignant cells within the pleural or peritoneal spaces, and with lymphatic obstruction. Lung and breast cancer are the most common causes of malignant pleural effusions, and the condition presents both diagnostic and therapeutic challenges. In this instance, the cause of the effusion is already known, and the diagnostic evaluation is limited.

3. Condition: Serious

3. Routine.

4. Allergies: NKA

4. Routine.

5. Vital Signs: Temp, BP, Pulse, Resp q.i.d.
Call physician if:
   Temp > 38.5°C
   BP < 90 systolic
   Resp > 30

5. Routine.

6. Activity: As tolerated

6. Routine.

7. Nursing: I and O × 24 h, otherwise routine measures

7. If a chest tube is required, an order should be written to place the chest tube through a water seal with constant suction.

8. Diet: House, no added salt

8. Routine.

9. IV Orders: None

9. Routine.

10. Medications:
Tamoxifen 10 mg PO b.i.d.
Routine:

10. The best treatment for malignant effusions is effective therapy against the offending

DOSS 250 mg PO qd
MOM 30 ml PO q hs prn for constipation
Triazolam 0.25 mg PO q hs prn for sleep
Meperidine 50 mg PO q 4 h prn for pain

11. Laboratory:
   Admission: CBC, PT, SMA-12, platelet count, CXR (PA and lateral with rt. lateral decubitus); send thoracentesis fluid for culture only; portable CXR (upright)—indication: post-thoracentesis

12. Special: Thoracentesis tray at bedside for therapeutic tap at 1600 hours

malignancy. In this instance, the patient was postmenopausal and had an estrogen-receptor positive breast cancer. Treatment with tamoxifen, an antiestrogen, was initiated.

11. Chest radiography can determine if fluid is loculated and can reveal pleural metastases. In addition, post-thoracentesis x-rays can indicate pneumothorax and reaccumulation of fluid.

12. The usual therapy for malignant effusions is to completely drain the effusion by thoracentesis and, if possible, institute some form of antitumor therapy. Previously inflamed pleurae may then adhere, obliterating the pleural space, or effective antitumor therapy may prevent reaccumulation. However, effusions commonly recur despite such therapy, and if this occurs, a low-lying chest tube is inserted, and the effusion is completely redrained.

   Once the effusion is completely drained and the visceral and parietal pleurae are in apposition, tetracycline for parenteral use (500 mg in 30 ml normal saline) may be infused through the tube, after which the tube is clamped. Over the next hour, the patient is positioned to assure that all free pleural surfaces are treated with the tetracycline. The chest tube is then removed. It should be noted that this type of tetracycline therapy is extremely painful, and the overall success rate is only about 50%. Some authorities recommend that its use be restricted to patients with respiratory compromise.

   According to some reports, bleomycin may be superior to tetracycline for pleurodesis.

Mucositis in Patients Receiving Chemotherapy

1. Admit: 6 Southeast

   1. Many large hospitals have oncology units, although a general medical ward would be another appropriate location for this patient.

2. Diagnosis: Mucositis

   2. Mucositis is a relatively common complication of many chemotherapeutic agents, usually occurring in mild form only. However, more severe mucositis occurs with radiotherapy to the head and neck, in bone marrow transplantation, or with higher doses of 5-FU, cyclophosphamide and several other agents. It occurs from a general inhibition of rapidly growing mucosal cells and is usually a diffuse process, most severe in the oral cavity. Patients are typically admitted when they are unable to take adequate fluids or control pain.

3. Condition: Stable

   3. Routine.

4. Allergies: NKA

   4. Routine.

5. Vital Signs: BP, Pulse, Resp, Temp q shift
   Call physician if:
   Temp > 38°C
   Pulse < 50, > 120/min
   BP < 90 systolic

   5. Infectious complications are common in this patient group and require prompt therapy.

6. Activity: Ad lib

   6. Routine.

7. Nursing care:
   Assist with mouth care as outlined below
   Strict handwashing
   I and O

   7. It is important to emphasize that handwashing to avoid nosocomial spread of infection is important in these patients.

8. Diet:
   Full liquids
   Supplemental per dietary recommendations

   8. In severe cases, parenteral nutrition will be necessary.

9. IV orders:
   #1. 1000 ml D5NS 200 ml/h
   #2. 1000 ml D5–½NS + 20 mEq KCl at 150 ml/h
   #3. 1000 ml D5–½NS + 20 mEq KCl at 150 ml/h

   9. Most patients will be volume depleted initially but able to maintain some oral intake. If not, they will need continuous intravenous support.

#4 Maintain heparin lock when IV fluids are finished

10. Medications:
Routine:
Acetaminophen 650 mg PO q 4 h
DOSS 250 mg PO t.i.d. with meals
Triazolam 0.25 mg PO q hs prn for sleep
Meperidine 50 mg–75 mg IV q 3 h prn for pain
Special Oral Care Regimen:
Normal saline rinses q 1 h
Viscous lidocaine 4%, rinse and spit (limit dose to 3 ml/h maximum)
Dyclonine 1% solution 15 ml with 15 mg diphenhydramine. Rinse and spit q 4 h prn for oral pain

10. If pain is severe, parenteral narcotics or a morphine drip may be necessary. Intravenous salicylates should be avoided, owing to the risk of bleeding.

Other empiric solutions to palliate oral pain include topical solutions of salicylates in saline and Rothwell's solution. Excessive use of lidocaine must be avoided.

11. Laboratory:
Admission: CBC, SMA-12 U/A, PT
Special: Culture oral cavity lesions for herpes simplex virus (HSV)

11. Other laboratory tests will be indicated based on patient's underlying tumor and other possible complications. For example, if the patient has a fever, sinus x-rays may be needed as well as a chest x-ray.

Cultures of the oral cavity are necessary, particularly for any ulcerated areas, because superinfection with herpes simplex virus is common and now treatable. If *Candida* or other opportunistic infections are suspected, appropriate cultures may also be indicated. Bleeding may also occur and coagulation parameters should be monitored.

12. Special:
Oral Medicine Service to see patient

12. In some patients, a consultation with either the ENT physicians or Oral Medicine Service may be helpful.

Pain

1. Admit to 8 South

1. Usually, patients are admitted to a general medicine floor or oncology unit.

2. Diagnosis: Lung cancer, metastatic to bone, severe pain

2. Patients with uncontrolled malignancy will commonly

develop severe, difficult-to-manage pain. On occasion, they require hospitalization for the management of pain and for general care. Such hospitalization can make the final days at home easier and more comfortable.

3. Condition: Serious

3. Routine.

4. Allergies: NKA

4. Routine.

5. Vital Signs: Temp, BP, Pulse, Resp q 8 h
Call physician if Temp > 38.5°C

5. In the care of the terminally ill, vital signs need not be taken frequently. However, these patients should not be ignored and left alone or made to feel deserted.

6. Activity: As tolerated

6. Routine.

7. Nursing:
Encourage patient to be up in a chair at least twice per shift, days and evenings; if patient stays in bed, turn at least twice per shift—sacral area is at risk for pressure ulcer; place an eggcrate mattress under the patient

7. The nursing staff can encourage as much activity as the patient can tolerate and provide consoling company. Bedsores are common in patients who have cachexia and are minimally active; every effort should be made to prevent their occurrence.

8. Diet: House; no restrictions

8. Routine.

9. IV Orders: None

9. Routine.

10. Medications:
Pain cocktail: Methadone, 8 mg, acetaminophen, 650 mg, and hydroxyzine, 50 mg, in 10 ml cherry syrup PO q 6 h
Routine:
Acetaminophen 650 mg PO q 4 h prn for Temp > 38°C
DOSS 250 mg PO qd
Triazolam 0.25 mg PO q hs prn for sleep
Morphine sulfate 5–10 mg PO or IM q 6 h prn for pain; call physician if patient asks for two consecutive doses in 6 hours or less

10. Pain can be treated in a variety of ways. A long-acting analgesic, such as methadone in a pain cocktail formula, has the advantages of requiring less frequent administration and maintaining fairly constant levels of analgesia and sedation. Other cocktails include amphetamine, antidepressants, and cocaine. Although the pain cocktail should keep the patient pain-free, an additional order for a prn narcotic will be helpful if the dose of methadone has been underestimated. Although meperidine is a popular narcotic for pain control, oral meperidine is not a very effective analgesic; oral morphine has become an increasingly popular option.

11. Laboratory: CBC, Ca⁺⁺, electrolytes, BUN, and glucose

11. For terminally ill patients, extensive laboratory studies serve little purpose.

12. Special: None

12. As indicated.

Spinal Cord Compression

1. Admit to 8 South

1. Patients are usually admitted to an oncology unit or general medicine floor.

2. Diagnosis: Metastatic prostate cancer, spinal cord compression

2. Spinal epidural metastases (especially from lung, breast, prostate, unknown primary tumors, and lymphomas) cause spinal cord compression in 5% of patients with disseminated malignant disease. Patients suffering from this complication generally have advanced cancer and a prognosis of short survival. Typical clinical manifestations of spinal cord compression are back pain exacerbated by recumbency, paraparesis, spinal sensory deficits, and sphincter dysfunction.

3. Condition: Serious

4. Allergies: NKA

5. Vital Signs: Temp, BP, Pulse, Resp q 8 h

6. Activity: Bed rest

7. Nursing
In and out bladder catheterization if patient fails to void during previous 8 hour shift. If residual is greater than 250 mg, then place Foley catheter and drain to gravity
I and O

7. Urinary retention may result from neurologic bladder paralysis or dysfunction.

8. Diet: House; no restrictions

9. IV Orders: D5W TKO

9. Certain patients may require intravenous hydration with D5NS if oral intake has been reduced by immobility.

10. Medications:
Dexamethasone 10 mg IV bolus now, then 4 mg IV or PO q 4 h

10. Immediate intervention is mandatory in spinal cord compression secondary to malignant disease, since progres-

Meperidine 50–75 mg IV/IM q 3 h prn for pain
DOSS 200 mg PO qd
Heparin 5000 units SC b.i.d.

sion can be rapid and neurologic recovery of lost function is unusual. Dexamethasone therapy is initiated immediately in any patient suspected of having neoplastic cord compression. Because back pain can be severe in these patients, adequate analgesia is important.

Because of the increased risk of DVT secondary to immobilization, subcutaneous heparin prophylaxis for DVT should be administered.

11. Laboratory:
Admission: CBC, SMA-12, UA

11. Routine.

12. Special:
MRI of the thoracic spine— R/O spinal cord compression in patient with metastatic prostate cancer and acute-onset bilateral lower-leg weakness (performed in ER)
Neurosurgery consultation
Medical oncology consultation
Radiation oncology consultation

12. MRI is now the preferred imaging method for detection and evaluation of spinal cord compression. If MRI is unavailable, then CT myelography should be performed. Any suspected spinal cord compression should be evaluated as soon as possible. The region of the cord compressed can often be predicted by the sensory level of neurologic impairment, if present. Radiation therapy is initiated promptly in patients with slow progression (weeks to months), incomplete block on MRI or myelography, radiosensitive tumors (e.g., lymphomas), or contraindications to major surgery. Patients with complete block on MRI or myelography, rapid progression, cervical compression, or an unknown primary tumor should undergo prompt decompressive laminectomy.

Thrombocytopenia and Anemia

1. Admit to 8 South

1. Patients are usually admitted to a general medicine floor.

2. Diagnosis: Testicular carcinoma, thrombocytopenia and anemia s/p chemotherapy

2. Thrombocytopenia can occur as a result of a disease process or from myelosuppressive

therapy. The thrombocytopenia and anemia in this case are primarily from chemotherapy, although the patient did have occult blood in his stools. Therapy for thrombocytopenia—platelet transfusion—is given at the first sign of bleeding or for platelet counts of less than 20,000/mm^3. Fatal hemorrhage usually occurs with platelet counts of less than 20,000/mm^3. Intracranial bleeding is a common terminal event.

3. Condition: Serious

3. The condition may be critical.

4. Allergies: NKA

4. Routine.

5. Vital Signs: Temp, BP, Pulse, Resp q 6 h
   Call physician if:
   Temp > 38.5°C
   BP < 90 systolic
   Pulse > 130
   Resp > 30

5. Taking vital signs monitors for the development of shock and sepsis.

6. Activity: Ad lib; avoid head or other bodily trauma; thrombocytopenic precautions

6. Every effort should be made to avoid trauma, which can lead to increased bleeding. Thrombocytopenic precautions are routine protocol in some hospitals.

7. Nursing:
   I and O
   No intramuscular injections
   No salicylates or salicylate-containing drugs

7. Routine.

8. Diet: House, with no caffeine-containing or alcoholic beverages

8. Routine.

9. IV Orders:
   Heparin lock; 2 units packed RBCs over 4 h; 6 units random donor platelets as soon as available

9. As noted previously, platelet transfusions (4–8 units per transfusion) are the treatment for chemotherapy-induced thrombocytopenia. Transfusion of red blood cells should be considered when the hematocrit is less than 25%, especially when there is evidence of bleeding and the possibility that it will be sustained bleeding.

10. Medications:
    Diphenhydramine 50 mg PO

10. Diphenhydramine is given to patients with a history of fe-

30 min before platelet transfusion

Ranitidine 150 mg PO b.i.d.

Routine:

DOSS 250 mg PO qd

MOM 30 ml PO q hs prn for constipation

Triazolam 0.25 mg PO q hs prn for sleep

Acetaminophen 650 mg PO q 4 h prn for Temp > 38°C

brile and urticarial reactions to the administration of platelets and blood products. Treatment with an H_2-blocker is used to minimize gastrointestinal blood loss. In females, contraceptives are commonly given to prevent menses during periods of marrow aplasia.

11. Laboratory:
Admission: CBC, platelet count, absolute polys, PT, PTT, fibrinogen, fibrinogen split products, electrolytes (already sent); arrange for CXR (PA and lateral), ECG, and platelet count 1 h after transfusion

Tomorrow: Hct, platelet count, absolute polys, K^+

11. A problem resulting from platelet transfusions is the production of platelet antibodies, which can develop rapidly in patients receiving multiple blood products. Failure to achieve a normal platelet increment at 1 hour (about 10,000/mm^3 per unit) in an afebrile patient should raise the suspicion that alloimmunization has occurred. In septic, febrile patients, platelet increments are much lower. Patients with bleeding should also be evaluated for the presence of DIC, but this is more commonly associated with generalized bleeding in the setting of sepsis or in certain patients with leukemia, especially acute promyelocytic leukemia and metastatic adenocarcinomas (of the prostate, pancreas, stomach).

12. Special: None

12. As indicated.

EXAMPLES OF ORDERS FOR IN-HOSPITAL CHEMOTHERAPY

Acute Myelogenous Leukemia

1. Admit to 8 South

1. Patients are usually admitted to a general medicine floor or oncology unit.

2. Diagnosis: Acute myelogenous leukemia, induction chemotherapy

2. This patient has been admitted for a course of induction chemotherapy, and the treatment follows a standard protocol for adult acute leukemia. A variety of protocols

exist for most malignancies that are managed with chemotherapy.

Each patient should be considered individually and an appropriate regimen designed with that patient in mind. This set of orders is based on an individual patient and is not appropriate for all patients.

3. Condition: Satisfactory

3. The patient may be in satisfactory condition at the beginning of chemotherapy or may be quite ill. Before chemotherapy every effort should be made to stabilize the patient by treatment of infections, rehydration, correction of electrolyte abnormalities, and transfusion with platelets and red blood cells as needed.

4. Allergies: NKA

4. Routine.

5. Vital Signs: Temp, BP, Pulse, Resp q 4 h; no rectal Temps
Daily weights
I and O
Call physician if:
   Temp > 38.5°C
   BP < 90 systolic
   Resp < 30

5. Taking vital signs monitors for the development of infection, volume depletion, and nutritional weight loss.

6. Activity: Ad lib

6. There is no need to restrict the patient's activity prior to the development of leukopenia. However, these patients are at risk for infection and should not have contact with obviously contagious persons. Furthermore, if the patient is thrombocytopenic, precautions must also be taken to avoid trauma, especially head trauma.

7. Nursing:
Teach patient proper mouth and rectal care
Encourage good PO intake
Start flow chart of daily maximum Temp, Hct, platelet count, WBC, polys, type of chemotherapy, date of chemotherapy, other medications, and transfusions
I and O

7. Proper mouth care is extremely important, since patients often develop mucositis, gingivitis, and oral candidiasis. Soothing mouth washes (with saline, antihistamine, or a local anesthetic such as viscous Xylocaine) and antifungal mouth washes such as nystatin suspension are helpful for these condi-

Test all urine for pH
Call physician if urine output
< 300 ml/4 h
No rectal Temps

8. Diet: House; encourage high caloric and fluid intake

9. IV Orders:
   #1–3. 1000 ml D5–½NS, with 1 amp NaHCO$_3$ (50 mEq), and 20 mEq KCl at 100 ml/h; repeat this IV solution × 2

10. Medications:
    Allopurinol 100 mg PO t.i.d.
    TMP-SMX double-strength tab (80 mg trimethoprim, 400 mg sulfamethoxazole)—1 tab PO b.i.d.
    Chemotherapy beginning tomorrow:
    Daunorubicin 100 mg IV every day on days 1, 2, and 3 (administer through a free-flowing IV that flows forward and returns blood easily; extravasation must be avoided)
    Cytosine arabinoside (Ara-C) 145 mg IV q 12 h on days 1, 2, 3, 4, 5, 6, 7, 8, 9
    Thioguanine 145 mg PO q 12 h on days 1, 2, 3, 4, 5, 6, 7, 8, 9

tions. In addition, diligent care must be taken of the rectal area, a common source of sepsis. Sitz baths can be used for this purpose.

A flow chart is indispensable in keeping track of the mass of clinical and laboratory data compiled on these complicated patients.

8. High fluid intake helps to maintain a high urine output and prevent volume depletion. Patients with a good nutritional status tolerate chemotherapy better and are less prone to infection.

9. Patients should be kept normovolemic, and every attempt should be made to maintain an adequate (75–100 ml/h) and alkaline urine output. The goal of IV therapy is to prevent the urate nephropathy to which patients with large tumor burdens are susceptible. Furosemide may be needed to maintain an adequate urine output; acetazolamide can be used to maintain an alkaline urine pH. Potassium losses may be profound in patients with leukemia.

10. Medication regimens may be complicated in patients receiving chemotherapy. Doses are calculated from existing protocols on the basis of the patient's body surface area. Drug toxicities are numerous, and clinicians must be familiar with the drugs they are administering.

The medications indicated here will not be reviewed in detail. However, it is important to note that anthracycline antibiotics (Adriamycin and daunorubicin) can cause severe local tissue necrosis if there is extravasation. Administration of dilute solutions through free-flowing IVs will minimize the chemical

Prednisone 20 mg PO t.i.d. on days 1, 2, 3, 4, 5, 6, 7, 8, 9

Vincristine 1.45 mg IV on days 1 and 9

Routine:

DOSS 250 mg PO q day

Flurazepam 30 mg PO q hs prn for sleep

Lorazepam 2 mg PO 30 min before chemotherapy

Metoclopramide 100 mg (2 mg/kg) and diphenhydramine 25 mg IV by slow infusion 30 min before each dose of daunorubicin, then 2 q h × 2

Droperidol 3 mg (2–5 mg) IV q 4 h prn for nausea

Acetazolamide 250 mg PO q 12 h prn for urine pH < 7

Normal saline or viscous Xylocaine mouthwash at bedside

Acetaminophen 650 mg PO q 4 h prn for Temp > 38°C

phlebitis resulting from these agents. In our hospital, daunorubicin is diluted in 50 ml of NS and administered through the side arm of a freely flowing IV. In many institutions, IV chemotherapy is conducted by physicians only.

Patients should be given allopurinol prior to chemotherapy and during the period of cell lysis. The drug should be discontinued when hypoplasia occurs.

Other routine medications include sedatives and antiemetics to counteract the effects of chemotherapy; antipyretics and analgesics, soothing mouthwashes, and drugs to alkalize the urine. Nystatin, clotrimazole troches, or amphotericin may be used for oral candidiasis. Trimethoprim-sulfa combination is given as a prophylactic antibiotic, especially for *Pneumocystis carinii*. The use of trimethoprim-sulfa is controversial in this setting.

11. Laboratory:

Admission: CBC with absolute polys, PT, platelet count, uric acid, SMA-12, HL-A typing (already sent)

Daily labs: Hct, WBC, platelet count, absolute polys, electrolytes, BUN, and glucose

11. Hematologic laboratory values are followed daily to monitor disease activity and the effects of chemotherapy and to plan transfusion and neutropenic therapy. The electrolyte levels are followed since abnormalities are common, especially hypokalemia, which can be severe. Patients receiving acetazolamide may develop metabolic acidosis.

12. Special: None now

12. As indicated.

Breast Cancer

1. Admit to 5 North

1. Most patients are admitted to a general medical or a specialized oncology unit.

2. Diagnosis: Metastatic breast cancer

2. Patients with breast cancer are admitted for treatment either because they develop

complications or when the chemotherapy regimen requires that the patients be inpatients. Many patients receive ongoing chemotherapy as outpatients. This patient was admitted to receive the standard CMF (cyclophosphamide, methotrexate, and 5-fluorouracil) regimen.

3. Condition: Stable

3. Routine.

4. Activity: Ad lib

4. Routine.

5. Vital signs: BP, Pulse, Temp, Resp q shift
   Call physician if:
   Pulse > 120
   Temp > 38°C
   BP < 100 systolic

5. Routine.

6. Allergies: NKA

6. Routine.

7. Nursing:
   I and O
   Daily weights
   Encourage PO intake
   Encourage ambulation
   Teaching: regarding breast cancer

7. Most patients will require IV hydration in addition to oral intake. Ambulation is important because patients with malignancies are at increased risk for deep venous thrombosis. A good teaching program is important and routine in many hospitals.

8. Diet: House; dietitian to encourage and monitor intake

8. Routine.

9. IV orders:
   #1. 1000 ml D5–½NS at 150 ml/h
   #2. 1000 ml D5–¼NS at 150 ml/h
   #3. Heparin lock; further IV orders to follow

9. Adequate hydration is essential. If intake is poor, then IV hydration should be continued to help prevent cystitis from cyclophosphamide. Many patients will become volume depleted from vomiting and poor intake.

10. Medications:
    Chemotherapy:
    Cyclophosphamide 100 mg PO days 1–14
    Methotrexate 35 mg IV day 1, day 8
    Fluorouracil 500 mg IV day 1, day 8
    Routine:
    DOSS 200 mg PO b.i.d.
    Lorazepam 2 mg PO 30 min prior to chemotherapy, days 1 and 8
    Prochlorperazine 5 mg IV q 4 h prn for nausea

10. The treatment for breast cancer depends on its stage, the age and menstrual status of the patient, as well as the hormone receptor status of the tumor. In this example, the patient is treated with the standard doses and medications for breast cancer. The doses are: cyclophosphamide 100 mg/m^2, methotrexate 35 mg/m^2, fluorouracil 500 mg/m^2. These drugs are usually administered every 4 weeks for 9–12 months. An

Diphenhydramine 50 mg PO q 4 h prn for nausea

If above medications ineffective for nausea, call physician

oncologist is usually involved in chemotherapy decisions. This patient was begun on chemotherapy in the hospital. However, not all patients will require inpatient chemotherapy with this particular regimen, and, in fact, this patient was able to leave the hospital after tolerating the first 3 days of therapy.

11. Laboratory
Admission: Chest x-ray, ECG, SMA-12, CBC
Tomorrow AM: BUN, electrolytes
Special studies:
Bone scan: indication—metastatic breast cancer

11. Electrocardiograms should be obtained in all patients who receive cyclophosphamide. Electrolytes should be carefully monitored in the early phases of therapy.

Bone scans are helpful if there is focal bone pain or an elevated alkaline phosphatase. A head CT scan or an abdominal CT scan may be indicated in some patients for assessment of liver or central nervous system metastases.

12. Special: None

12. Routine.

Germ Cell Tumor

1. Admit to 6 Southeast

1. General medical floors or specialized oncology units are appropriate. If the tumor load is large, the patient is at risk for tumor lysis syndrome and may need ICU monitoring.

2. Diagnosis: Germ cell tumor

2. A variety of germ cell tumors exist; the therapy varies according to the type of tumor.

3. Condition: Satisfactory

3. Patients with germ cell tumors are usually in satisfactory condition and are less likely than patients with hematologic malignancy to have developed early complications.

4. Allergies: NKA

4. Routine.

5. Vital Signs: BP, Pulse, Temp, Resp q shift
Call physician if:
BP < 90 systolic
Pulse > 120
Temp > 38°C

5. Monitoring for fever is essential, although the neutropenia associated with therapy usually occurs 1–14 days after therapy.

6. Activity: Ad lib

6. Restriction is to be discouraged—patients should remain as active as possible.

7. Nursing:
Encourage PO intake
I and O
Teaching: Mouth care, neutropenic precautions

7. Good teaching is of utmost importance early in the course of treatment, both for patient understanding to allay fear and to help the patient become alert to complications.

8. Diet: Routine, encourage >2000 kcal/day

8. Maintenance of nutritional status is important, especially for long-term therapy.

9. IV orders:
#1. 1000 ml D5–½NS at 200 ml/h
#2. 1000 ml D5–½NS at 150 ml/h
#3. 1000 ml D5–½NS at 150 ml/h
Further orders to be written daily; check with physician if necessary

9. Younger patients will usually tolerate vigorous hydration. This will lower the risk of complications associated with *cis*-platinum treatment. Vigorous hydration will also minimize complications associated with tumor lysis syndrome, a problem of particular importance during initial therapy of bulky tumors.

10. Medications:
Chemotherapy:
Vinblastine 5 mg/m^2 IV first day only
Bleomycin 30 U IV q week
cis-Platinum (CDDP) 20 mg/m^2 IV days 1–5
Etoposide 100 mg/m^2 IV days 1–5
Antiemetics:
Lorazepam 2 mg PO 30 min before chemotherapy
Metoclopramide 0.5 mg/kg IV q 2 h for 6 doses; begin 30 min prior to chemotherapy
Diphenhydramine 50 mg IV 30 min prior to chemotherapy
Routine: DOSS 250 mg PO t.i.d. with meals
Triazolam 0.25 mg PO q hs prn for sleep
Acetaminophen 650 mg PO q 4 h prn for pain

10. This is a standard chemotherapy regimen for a germ cell tumor. The limiting factor in many chemotherapy protocols is acceptance by patients, owing to the side effects of nausea and vomiting, especially with chemotherapy protocols including *cis*-platinum. There are at least six agents that can be used for antiemetics: lorazepam, metoclopramide, diphenhydramine, dexamethasone, prochlorperazine, and tetrahydrocannabinol (THC). Usually one or two of these agents is effective. With regimens containing *cis*-platinum, it is wise to attempt a more vigorous protocol. In this case, the physician has ordered a particularly potent set of medications providing both sedation and antinausea/antiemetic effect. THC is occasionally of use, but a special permit is required.
   If the tumor load is particularly large, a "tumor lysis" syndrome may occasionally occur. Patients at risk for this

syndrome should be treated with allopurinol and phosphate binders before chemotherapy is initiated.

11. Laboratory:
Today: CBC, SMA-12
Tomorrow AM: BUN, creatinine, electrolytes

11. Routine chest x-ray and ECG are unnecessary after they have been obtained for use as a baseline. Electrolytes must be carefully monitored anytime *cis*-platinum is used. If the chemotherapy regimen places the patient at risk for myelosuppression, the CBC will need to be followed when the chemotherapy bone marrow suppression effect is at its peak.

12. Special: None

12. Routine.

Oat Cell Carcinoma

1. Admit to 6 Southeast

1. Most patients are admitted to a general medical floor or to a specialized oncology unit.

2. Diagnosis: Small cell cancer of the lung

2. Small cell or oat cell cancer of the lung accounts for 15% to 20% of lung cancers. Most are disseminated by the time of diagnosis, but a few patients have localized disease that completely responds to concurrent or rapidly alternating chemotherapy and chest irradiation and is potentially curable. Whole-brain irradiation is used by most centers as prophylaxis against relapse at that site in patients who achieve remission.

3. Condition: Serious

3. Most patients are systemically ill by the time of diagnosis.

4. Allergies: NKA

4. Routine.

5. Activity: Ad lib

5. Routine.

6. Vital Signs: BP, Pulse, Temp, Resp q shift
Call physician if
BP < 90 systolic
Temp > 38.5°C
Resp > 30

6. Routine. Fever may be seen with postobstructive pneumonia or when bone marrow involvement occurs.

7. Nursing:
   Daily weights
   I and O
   Encourage PO intake
   Please make flow chart of daily labs

7. Careful monitoring of input and output is necessary to assure an adequate volume status. Patients may be extremely cachectic and have little reserve. An orderly flow sheet is of considerable value in patients undergoing a rigorous chemotherapy protocol.

8. Diet: House

8. If oral intake is poor and nutritional stores are inadequate, some form of supplemental alimentation may be necessary.

9. IV Orders:
   #1. 1000 ml D5–½NS + 20 mEq KCl at 200 ml/h
   #2. 1000 ml D5–½NS + 20 mEq KCl at 150 ml/h
   #3. 1000 ml D5–½NS + 20 mEq KCl at 150 ml/h

9. Patients receiving large doses of cyclophosphamide must receive adequate IV hydration. This is generally true for most patients receiving chemotherapy. Doxorubicin (Adriamycin) must be administered in a free-flowing IV to minimize risk of extravasation.

10. Medications:
    Chemotherapy:
    Vincristine 2 mg IV day 1
    Doxorubicin (Adriamycin) 75 mg IV day 1
    Cyclophosphamide 1100 mg IV day 1
    Antiemetics:
    Diphenhydramine 50 mg IV q 4 h prn for nausea and vomiting
    Metoclopramide 20 mg IV q 6 h prn for nausea and vomiting
    Prochlorperazine 5 mg IV q 4 h prn for nausea and vomiting
    Routine:
    DOSS 100 mg PO b.i.d. with meals
    Acetaminophen 650 mg PO q 4 h prn for pain
    MOM 30 ml PO q hs prn if no stool that day

10. There are several protocols for small cell carcinoma, although the response is not significantly different from the standard "VAC" regimen listed above. The dose of doxorubicin is 50 mg/m^2 and that for cyclophosphamide is 750 mg/m^2. An alternative is a VP-16, *cis*-platinum combination. The VAC regimen is repeated on a monthly basis and adjustments may be made based on neutrophil and platelet counts following chemotherapy. As with other chemotherapy regimens, an oncologist should be involved with decisions regarding administration of chemotherapeutic agents.

Many antiemetic regimens may be used. The patient and the nursing staff together will generally find a regimen that is most effective in that particular case. Diphenhydramine may help counteract the extrapyramidal side effects seen with both metoclopramide and prochlorperazine.

11. Laboratory:
    Admission: ECG, chest x-ray, PT, CBC, SMA-12
    Tomorrow: BUN, electrolytes
    Special Studies:
    Schedule CT scan of head and upper abdomen—indication: small cell lung cancer
    Schedule bone scan—indication: small cell lung cancer

11. A chest x-ray may not be needed if a recent film is available. Electrolytes must be monitored carefully in patients receiving chemotherapy and IV hydration.

    Staging of small cell carcinoma usually involves examination of the central nervous system, bone marrow, and liver to assess whether the disease is limited or extensive.

12. Special: Bone marrow aspiration and biopsy to be performed this afternoon at 3 PM (1500 h). Please arrange for bone marrow tray to be ready at that time

12. Examination of the marrow is frequently included in staging for small cell carcinoma.

NEUROLOGIC DISEASES

ALCOHOL WITHDRAWAL

1. Admit to 6 North

   1. Usually, patients are admitted to a general medicine or neurology service.

2. Diagnosis: Alcohol withdrawal, s/p seizure

   2. The major manifestations of the alcohol withdrawal or abstinence syndrome are tremulousness, hallucinosis, seizures, and delirium. Mild forms of the syndrome (tremulousness, hallucinations, seizures, or "rum fits") are generally easy to manage and must be distinguished from delirium tremens, a life-threatening illness that requires a different management approach. This patient was admitted after a seizure with tremulousness and hallucinosis.

3. Condition: Satisfactory

   3. Routine.

4. Allergies: NKA

   4. Routine.

5. Vital Signs: Temp, Pulse, BP, Resp q 4 h
   Call physician if:
   BP < 90 systolic
   Temp > 38.5°C
   Pulse > 130

   5. Taking vital signs helps to monitor the patient for the development of the increased autonomic activity characteristic of delirium tremens and for signs of infection. "DTs" are distinguished from the milder forms of withdrawal by the presence of fever, tachycardia, profuse sweating, profound confusion, delusions, vivid, frightening hallucinations, tremor, agitation, and sleeplessness.

6. Activity: Bed rest with bathroom privileges; up in a chair

   6. Routine.

7. Nursing:
   Call physician for increase in confusion, hallucination, agitation, and tremor
   Seizure precautions

   7. Nurses should observe the patient for symptoms and signs of DTs, so that appropriate therapy can be instituted.

8. Diet: House

   8. Routine.

9. IV Orders: None

   9. In mild withdrawal, IV therapy is not required unless the patient is volume-depleted. However, in delirium tremens, IV therapy is essential for the administration of

fluids and for the correction of electrolyte depletion, especially for losses of sodium, potassium, and magnesium. Volume depletion in severe cases may require the administration of 6 liters of fluid daily.

10. Medications:
    Thiamine 100 mg PO qd
    Folate 1 mg PO qd
    Chlordiazepoxide 50 mg IM now, then 50 mg IM or PO q 6 h prn for agitation or hallucination

10. Thiamine is given routinely to alcoholics to prevent the precipitation of Wernicke-Korsakoff encephalopathy. Most alcoholics are also folate-deficient and can be treated for this. Treatment of the symptoms of alcohol withdrawal is usually accomplished with benzodiazepines (diazepam, lorazepam, chlordiazepoxide), or phenobarbital. Beta-blockers and clonidine may also be used.

    The term "seizure" usually refers to a single seizure or a few separate seizures occurring in a short time. Anticonvulsants are not indicated unless the patient has an underlying seizure disorder.

11. Laboratory:
    Admission: CBC, PT, SMA-12, Mg, UA, CXR, ECG

11. Laboratory studies to evaluate the patient for anemia and electrolyte disturbance are important. In patients with delirium tremens, a careful search should be made for underlying infection.

12. Special: Social work consult

12. Special referrals must be made on an individual basis; social workers are best trained to make appropriate referrals.

DRUG ADDICTION

1. Admit to 6 West

1. Usually, patients are admitted to a general medicine or neurology service.

2. Diagnosis: Cellulitis, lt. arm; narcotic addiction

2. Narcotic addicts are admitted to the hospital for a variety of medical and surgical crises. Attempts to withdraw the addict from opiates during an acute illness complicates the management of these ill-

nesses and are unlikely to be successful. Therefore, patients should be treated for their acute illness, and decisions about withdrawal should be postponed until that phase of the illness is over.

Two types of addicts are commonly admitted, i.e., those in methadone maintenance programs and "street addicts" who admit to or have demonstrated evidence of addiction but who are not enrolled in a drug abuse program. This patient was admitted for cellulitis related to the injection of narcotics and was a known street addict.

3. Condition: Satisfactory

3. Routine.

4. Allergies: NKA; pentazocine is not to be given

4. Addicts should not be given pentazocine, which, as a narcotic antagonist, may precipitate a withdrawal reaction in an opiate-dependent patient.

5. Vital Signs: Temp, BP, Pulse, Resp q 6 h
   Call physician if:
   Temp > 39°C
   BP < 90 or > 180 systolic
   Pulse > 130

5. Taking vital signs monitors the patient for signs of withdrawal and the progress of infection.

6. Activity: Keep lt. arm elevated, otherwise no restriction

6. Routine.

7. Nursing:
   Warm soaks to area of cellulitis t.i.d.
   Observe for withdrawal symptoms and chart:
   Grade I: lacrimation, rhinorrhea, diaphoresis, yawning, restlessness, insomnia
   Grade II: Dilated pupils, piloerection, muscle twitching, myalgia, arthralgia, abdominal pain
   Grade III: Tachycardia, hypertension, tachypnea, fever, anorexia, nausea, restlessness

7. The nursing staff can observe the patient for signs of withdrawal and alert the clinician to the need for repeated evaluation or more narcotic.

Grade IV: Diarrhea, vomiting, postural hypotension, curled-up position

8. Diet: House

8. Routine.

9. IV Orders: None

9. Routine.

10. Medications:
Nafcillin 1.5 g IV q 6 h
Methadone 10 mg PO qd
Clonidine 0.1 mg PO t.i.d.
If withdrawal symptoms are observed, call physician, then give:
Methadone 5.0 mg PO qd for Grade I
Methadone 10.0 mg PO qd for Grade II
Methadone 15.0 mg PO qd for Grade III
Methadone 20.0 mg PO qd for Grade IV
Give morphine 3 mg SC at the same time as methadone for withdrawal
Routine:
DOSS 250 mg PO qd
MOM 30 ml PO q hs prn for constipation
Triazolam 0.25 mg PO q hs prn for sleep

10. Periodic use of a narcotic should not be equated with addiction. Therefore care must be exercised in initiating methadone treatment to avoid addicting a person to methadone who is not already dependent. In this instance, the patient was a well-known addict with obvious needle tracks. Therefore, he was given a modest dose of methadone to forestall withdrawal symptoms. The sliding scale has been devised for patients in whom withdrawal symptoms are observed and allows for the estimation of the initial methadone dose. A short-acting narcotic such as morphine is given with methadone because the oral administration of methadone usually takes from 2–4 hours to have any significant effect. Clonidine is used to suppress the autonomic "rebound" phenomenon that occurs during opiate withdrawal.

11. Laboratory:
Admission: Blood cultures × 2, CXR (PA and lateral), CBC, SMA-12, UA, culture and Gram stain of exudate from needle track (done)

11. Routine.

12. Special: Social work consult

12. Consultation with a social worker will provide the patient with treatment options.

PARKINSON'S DISEASE

1. Admit to 6 North

1. Usually, patients are admitted to a general medicine or neurology service.

2. Diagnosis: Parkinson's disease

2. Patients with Parkinson's disease are usually admitted to

the hospital because of some other illness. Occasionally, however, patients are admitted to begin medical therapy of Parkinson's disease and to plan comprehensive care. This elderly man had severe symptoms and was admitted to begin therapy with L-dopa and to plan a program for his wife to help care for him.

3. Condition: Satisfactory

3. Routine.

4. Allergies: NKA

4. Routine.

5. Vital Signs: Temp, BP, Pulse, Resp q shift; postural BP and Pulse every day
Call physician if:
Temp > 38.5°C
BP < 90 systolic

5. Postural hypotension is common in such patients and may be exacerbated by drug therapy.

6. Activity: Up with assistance only, as tolerated; up in a chair for meals

6. Inactivity, tremor, and rigidity are characteristics of patients with Parkinson's disease. Patients should initially be assisted with activities in the hope that they will eventually become more independent.

7. Nursing:
Assist patient with self-care and personal hygiene
Encourage patient to walk around room and in hall b.i.d.

7. Patients may need much encouragement to get them moving.

8. Diet: House

8. Routine.

9. IV Orders: None

9. Routine.

10. Medications:
Amantadine HCl 100 mg PO qd
Carbidopa 25 mg and levodopa 100 mg (combination) PO q 8 h
Routine:
DOSS 250 mg PO qd
MOM 30 ml PO q hs prn for constipation
Triazolam 0.25 mg PO q hs prn for sleep, may repeat once

10. L-Dopa has become the cornerstone of drug therapy for Parkinson's disease. It is now given with carbidopa, an inhibitor of peripheral decarboxylation of levodopa. Amantadine is an antiviral agent that is a less potent antiparkinsonian drug than L-dopa but that may be helpful when given in addition to L-dopa. L-Dopa therapy is initiated at low doses and then increased gradually, and the patient is monitored for side effects and therapeutic efficacy.

11. Laboratory:
    Admission: CBC, SMA-12, UA, CXR (PA and lateral), ECG

11. Routine.

12. Special:
    Physical therapy: General exercise and walking program
    Occupational therapy: Assessment of and help with daily home activities
    PT and OT to see wife and patient together, please

12. PT and OT consultations may be quite helpful for both patient and family.

SEIZURES

1. Admit to 5 South

1. Usually, patients are admitted to a general medicine or neurology service. Patients who have been treated for status epilepticus in the ER should be admitted to the ICU.

2. Diagnosis: Recurrent seizures, postictal state

2. It is worthwhile to indicate if the patient has recurrent seizures or is being admitted after an initial seizure.

3. Condition: Satisfactory

3. The condition of patients with status epilepticus should be considered serious or critical, depending on the etiology.

4. Allergies: NKA

4. Routine.

5. Vital Signs: Temp, BP, Pulse, Resp q 4 h for 24 h, then q 6 h; neurologic checks q 4 h for 24 h
   Call physician if:
   BP < 80 systolic
   Temp > 39° C
   Pulse > 120
   Resp > 30

5. Routine.

6. Activity: As tolerated

6. Routine.

7. Nursing:
   Observe patient as frequently as possible; bed rails up, padded tongue blade at bedside

7. If it is convenient, patients with seizures may be placed in observation rooms or in the hall until it is certain that seizure activity is under control.

8. Diet: NPO until alert, then house diet

8. Routine.

9. IV Orders: Heparin lock

9. It is important to maintain an IV route.

10. Medications:
    Phenytoin 100 mg PO t.i.d.
    Phenobarbital 30 mg PO q.i.d.
    Triazolam 0.25 mg PO q hs
    prn for sleep
    MOM 30 ml PO q hs prn for
    constipation
    Special: Continue mainte-
    nance dose of seizure medi-
    cations

10. The patient's usual antisei-
    zure medications should be
    continued. The usual pheny-
    toin (Dilantin) dose is
    300–500 mg/day, and the
    usual dose of phenobarbital is
    90–210 mg/day. If rapid ad-
    ministration of phenytoin is
    required, 1000 mg may be
    given IV at the rate of 50
    mg/min (do not mix with
    D5W). Phenytoin should pref-
    erably be given slowly, di-
    rectly through the heparin
    lock. Administration of phen-
    ytoin by mouth may be
    achieved by giving 500 mg
    with a repeat 500 mg dose 12
    hours later, then giving a
    maintenance dose the follow-
    ing day.

11. Laboratory:
    Admission: CBC with differ-
    ential, SMA-12, UA, CXR
    (PA and lateral), phenytoin
    and phenobarbital levels

11. Patients under 40 years of age
    do not need a routine ECG
    unless cardiac disease is sus-
    pected. Obtaining drug levels
    is useful to determine if the
    seizure has occurred because
    of inadequate drug coverage
    (due usually to poor medica-
    tion compliance).

12. Special:
    Arrange EEG and include
    sleep periods—indication:
    Recurrent seizures after
    one year of good control

12. If the patient shows focal neu-
    rologic findings during a sei-
    zure or the interictal period or
    on EEG, a CT scan should be
    considered. CTs are almost al-
    ways done as part of a first
    seizure work-up. An LP
    should be done if meningitis
    or subarachnoid bleeding is
    suspected.

ALZHEIMER'S-TYPE DEMENTIA

1. Admit to 5 South

1. Usually, patients are admitted to a general medicine or
   neurology service.

2. Diagnosis: Confusion, agitation, probable Alzheimer's-
   type dementia

2. Patients are admitted to the
   hospital for the management
   of confusion and complications of dementia or for diagnostic evaluation. In all cases,
   a careful evaluation should be
   made of the underlying cause

for confusion or of conditions that might exacerbate the confusion in a patient with dementia of known cause. This patient was an elderly man with confusion of 2 years' duration who became increasingly agitated and confused and was admitted for evaluation.

3. Condition: Satisfactory

3. Routine.

4. Allergies: NKA

4. Routine.

5. Vital Signs: Temp, BP, Pulse, Resp q.i.d.; postural BP and Pulse qd
   Call physician if:
   Temp > 38.5°C
   BP < 90 systolic

5. Routine.

6. Activity: Ad lib, but restrict to ward

6. Patients with dementia tend to wander and become lost. In general, they need not be restrained (which may make them more agitated), but they should be restricted to some specific area.

7. Nursing:
   Attempt to reassure and reorient the patient when confused and agitated

7. Good nursing skills are needed to deal with the patient's agitation and confusion, which can be difficult to manage and tolerate. Reassurance, prevention of sudden stresses and changes, and consistent responses to patient demands may be helpful.

8. Diet: House

8. Routine.

9. IV Orders: None

9. Routine.

10. Medications:
    Haloperidol 0.5–1 mg PO q 4–8 h prn for agitation, not to exceed 4.0 mg/day
    DOSS 250 mg PO qd

10. In general, sedatives should not be used in elderly patients with organic brain syndrome. The side effects of medications, especially sedatives, are perhaps the most common causes of confusion in the elderly. However, low doses of a drug such as haloperidol may be necessary at times. It is wise to start with low doses in patients with dementia, who can be extraordinarily sensitive to psychotropic drugs. Higher doses can be given if needed.

11. Laboratory:
    Admission: CBC, ESR, SMA-12 T4, T3RU, B-12, VDRL, UA, CXR (PA and lateral), ECG, and CT brain scan

11. The purpose of the laboratory evaluation of a patient with dementia of unknown cause is to determine if there are other causes of the dementia, such as myxedema, subdural hematoma, or giant-cell arteritis.

12. Special: Social worker to see wife and family to assist with home or chronic hospital care

12. Families may need help in planning for the long-term care of their disabled relative. Some patients and families may benefit from specialized dementia clinics designed to address the multiple needs of these patients and their families.

STROKE SYNDROME

1. Admit to 5 South

1. Usually, patients are admitted to a general medicine or neurology service.

2. Diagnosis: Stroke syndrome, rt. hemiparesis, ? aphasia

2. If possible, focal findings should be listed, e.g., "right hemiparesis."

3. Condition: Serious

3. The patient's condition will vary, depending on the severity of the stroke.

4. Allergies: NKA

4. Routine.

5. Vital Signs: Temp, BP, Pulse, Resp q 4 h for 24 h, then q 6 h
   Call physician if:
   BP < 80 or > 180 systolic or > 120 diastolic
   Temp > 39°C
   Pulse > 120
   Resp > 30
   Neurologic checks q 1 h for 12 h, then q 2 h for 12 h, then q 4 h; call physician for abrupt changes in neurologic status

5. Neurologic checks vary from hospital to hospital, but they usually include checks of pupillary size, level of consciousness, respiratory rate, and motor function (e.g., ability to grip; obviously if the leg is involved, motor strength in the leg should be checked). If consciousness is not impaired, neurologic checks can be done less frequently. The respiratory rate should be checked often in patients with brain stem strokes.

6. Activity: As tolerated, with assistance only; up in a chair t.i.d.

6. Activity orders have to be individualized according to the patient's motor and sensory deficits. There is no reason to restrict the patient to bed if he or she can ambulate.

7. Nursing:
   Turn patient frequently when awake
   Air mattress and sheepskin on bed
   Heel and elbow pads on rt. side
   Approach patient from lt. side, if possible

7. Special nursing orders should be tailored to each patient. For example, if the patient is hemiparetic, the nursing staff should be instructed to approach from the unaffected side. The patient should be positioned so that the doorway is on the "good" side.

8. Diet: House, as tolerated; assist with feeding

8. Often, patients with brain stem infarcts cannot swallow well and should be given soft or puréed foods.

9. IV Orders: None

9. Maintenance IV fluids will be required if the patient is unable to eat or drink.

10. Medications:
    DOSS 250 mg PO qd
    MOM 30 ml PO q hs prn for constipation

10. If the patient's level of consciousness is changing, the use of hypnotics and sedatives should be avoided.

    In some institutions, dexamethasone is given to stroke patients, especially if a substantial amount of brain tissue is infarcted. If herniation of the brain stem occurs, the patient should receive mannitol, 1.5 g/kg IV over 20–30 minutes; this may be repeated q 2 h prn. Frequent administration of mannitol may lead to volume depletion or hypernatremia or both. Hypertension often accompanies acute stroke and frequently is self-limited. The treatment is controversial, but it is probably indicated if the diastolic blood pressure is > 120 mm Hg. Therapy should not be too aggressive; an attempt should be made to lower the diastolic blood pressure to 90–100 mm Hg. Gradual lowering of blood pressure is probably better than precipitating an abrupt fall.

11. Laboratory:
    Admission: CBC with differential, PT, SMA-12, UA, CXR (PA and lateral), ECG

11. A small percentage of patients with strokes have acute myocardial infarctions. Causes of stroke that are nonatherosclerotic should be considered in all patients, but especially in younger patients; these

causes include leukemia, sickle cell anemia, polycythemia, and autoimmune disease with vasculitis.

12. Special:
Physical therapist to see patient for passive and active range of motion exercises

12. A CT scan should be ordered if there is a diagnostic question of subdural or subarachnoid bleeding, tumor, or abscess. Other studies that can be done if there are diagnostic problems include MRI, LP, EEG, and cerebral arteriography. In this patient, the presentation was so typical that further evaluation was not pursued.

SUBARACHNOID HEMORRHAGE

1. Admit to 5 South

1. Patients are usually admitted to a neurosurgery, neurology, or general medicine service.

2. Diagnosis: Subarachnoid hemorrhage, rt. arm weakness

2. Indicate the presence of focal neurologic signs. This patient has focal signs on the right side.

3. Condition: Serious

3. Obtunded or comatose patients should be considered critically ill.

4. Allergies: NKA

4. Routine

5. Vital Signs: Temp, BP, Pulse, Resp q 2 h for 12 h, then q 4 h for 12 h, then q 6 h
Call physician if:
BP < 80 systolic
Temp > 39°C
Pulse > 120
Resp > 30
Neurologic checks q 1 h for 12 h, then q 2 h for 12 h, then q 4 h; call physician for abrupt changes in neurologic status

5. If consciousness is not impaired, neurologic checks can be done less frequently.

6. Activity: Strict bed rest

6. Strict bed rest should be maintained for the first several days. A bedside commode may be allowed at the discretion of the physician.

7. Nursing:
Restrict visitors to visiting hours; may visit no more

7. Many physicians restrict visitors routinely to minimize the stimulation to the patient,

than 15 minutes, 2 visits per hour, 2 visitors at a time

8. Diet: Restrict total fluids to 1000 ml/day; remainder of diet as tolerated (if possible, should be high-residue with prunes)

9. IV Orders: Heparin lock

10. Medications:
Special:
Phenytoin 500 mg PO, STAT, and 500 mg PO in AM; 300 mg PO q AM thereafter
Nimodipine 60 mg q 4 h
Dexamethasone 10 mg PO, STAT, and 4 mg PO q 6 h
Routine:
MOM 30 ml PO q hs prn if no stool that day
DOSS 100 mg PO q.i.d.

11. Laboratory:
Admission: CBC with differential, PT, SMA-12, UA, CXR (portable AP), ECG

12. Special:
CT scan—indication: suspected anterior communicating aneurysm with hemorrhage
LP tray at bedside after CT scan
Consultation with neurosurgeon (already called)

but good judgment is required.

8. Fluids are restricted to maintain a state of relative volume depletion.

9. IV fluids (a total of 1000–1500 ml/day) are needed if the patient cannot eat or drink. The heparin lock is in place if mannitol is required.

10. The use of hypnotics and sedatives should be avoided if the patient's consciousness is altered. Many patients with subarachnoid hemorrhage have seizures, and antiseizure therapy is helpful. Steroids are sometimes given to reduce meningeal irritation, but the use of these drugs is controversial. Nimodipine, a calcium channel blocker, is used to reduce the severity of neurologic deficits resulting from vasospasm.

Aminocaproic acid (Amicar) is sometimes used to prevent lysis of the clot and thus to reduce the likelihood of rebleeding. Amicar has significant side effects and should be given only by physicians who have experience using the drug.

Stools should be kept soft and bowel movements should be regular to avoid straining, which could raise intracranial pressure.

11. ST- and T-wave changes and syndrome of inappropriate ADH secretion (SIADH) may be seen in patients with subarachnoid hemorrhage.

12. Three-vessel cerebral arteriography is usually done in the first several days of hospitalization. Early neurosurgical consultation is of critical importance.

SUSPECTED METASTASES TO THE CENTRAL NERVOUS SYSTEM (CNS)

1. Admit to ICU

1. If a CNS lesion is suspected, careful observation for herniation is necessary.

2. Diagnosis: Metastatic carcinoma, brain metastasis

2. Carcinoma of the breast and lung, as well as malignant melanoma, commonly metastasize to the brain.

3. Condition: Critical

3. After observation for 24 hours, the condition can be upgraded to serious if the patient improves.

4. Allergies: NKA

4. Routine.

5. Vital Signs: BP, Pulse, Temp, Resp q 1 h per ICU routine Neuro signs q 15 min × 4, then q 1 h × 12

5. Careful checks for development of focal findings are of utmost importance. If detected, they are a medical emergency and demand immediate therapy.

6. Activity: Strict bed rest

6. Routine.

7. Nursing:
   Routine flow charting, I and O; see neuro checks

7. The major nursing task in the first 12 to 24 hours is to monitor the patient for development of neurologic worsening.

8. Diet: NPO

8. Routine.

9. IV orders: 500 ml D5W, TKO for 24 h

9. Attempts are often made to induce intravascular volume depletion in the hopes of decreasing brain swelling. Intravenous fluids should initially be limited to medications and those required to ensure an open IV line.

10. Medications:
    Dexamethasone 10 mg IV now, then 6 mg IV q 6 h
    Furosemide 20 mg IV now
    Mannitol 100 g; keep available at bedside at all times
    Routine: None

10. The primary treatment of brain edema is intravenous steroid therapy. Mannitol should be available for immediate use in case of acute deterioration; if mannitol is used, the serum osmolality must be monitored carefully.

11. Laboratory:
    Admission: CBC, SMA-12, PT, UA, portable CXR, ECG
    Special Study: CT scan, STAT

11. At present, the standard of practice is to obtain a CT scan prior to performing a lumbar puncture if the latter is necessary to evaluate for possible infection. The CT scan will usually confirm the presence

12. Special: Intubation tray at the bedside; neurosurgical and radiotherapy consults today

12. or absence of focal metastases.

    If deterioration occurs and patient survival is anticipated, the patient can be treated with hyperventilation, thereby acutely lowering the CNS edema transiently while other therapy is pursued. The primary treatment of CNS metastasis remains radiotherapy, although surgery may be the procedure of choice in certain instances (for example, posterior fossa tumors, large tumors of the cortex with impending herniation, and so forth).

RENAL DISEASES

CHRONIC RENAL FAILURE AND HYPERKALEMIA

1. Admit to the ICU

1. Patients may be admitted to the ICU, a medical floor, or a dialysis unit.

2. Diagnosis: Chronic renal failure, hyperkalemia, hypertension

2. Chronically diseased kidneys can support life in reasonable comfort until 90% of the glomerular filtration rate (GFR) is lost. However, as filtration rates decline, the kidneys lose their ability to regulate concentrations of water, sodium, potassium, phosphate, magnesium, and other solutes and to maintain normal body fluid homeostasis. In this particular patient, who has chronic renal failure on the basis of long-standing hypertension, the injudicious use of spironolactone for edema resulted in dangerously serious hyperkalemia (K^+ of 7.0 mEq/100 ml), necessitating hospitalization. Normally, this patient managed well without dialysis, as do many others, and had a GFR of 20 ml/minute on antihypertensive therapy with moderate sodium, potassium, and water restriction.

3. Condition: Critical

3. Routine.

4. Allergies: NKA

4. Routine.

5. Vital Signs: ICU routine: BP, Pulse, Resp, cardiac monitor checks q 1 h; Temp q 4 h
   Call physician if:
   BP < 90 systolic
   Pulse > 120 or < 60
   VT, or QRS complex > 0.14 sec
   Daily weights

5. Arrhythmias are the most serious complication of hyperkalemia. For this reason, patients with severe hyperkalemia are managed in the CCU or ICU, where constant monitoring is available.

6. Activity: Bed rest for now

6. Routine.

7. Nursing:
   I and O q 2 h
   Insert Foley catheter if no urine output for 4 h

7. Monitoring the urine output is essential in this instance. If possible, Foley catheterization or any instrumentation in patients with renal failure should be avoided. However, catheterization may be re-

149

8. Diet: 80 mEq Na^+ and 60 g protein; no potassium-containing salt substitutes

9. IV Orders:
$NaHCO_3$ 50 mEq IV over 5 min, STAT
200 ml D50W with 10 U regular insulin at 50 ml/h
Call physician for next IV order after repeat K^+ level is available

10. Medications:
Polystyrene sulfonate (Kayexalate) 30 g (2 tsp) in 100 ml 20% sorbitol solution PO now and in 4 h
Hold all other medications (propranolol, multivitamins, DOSS, aluminum hydroxide gel) until tomorrow, when further orders will be written

11. Laboratory:
Admission: Electrolytes, ABGs, creatinine, BUN, Ca^{++}, CBC, STAT; UA, urine Gram stain and C and S, Mg^{++}, phosphate, uric acid, CXR (portable AP), ECG
Electrolytes, STAT; again in 3 h

quired to adequately monitor urine output.

8. Because the kidney has a limited ability to excrete sodium, potassium, and protein breakdown products, limits on the dietary intake of these substances are often required. Dietary restrictions are written in mEq or in grams of sodium and grams of protein.

9. The correction of acidosis and glucose and insulin infusion will cause potassium to move intracellularly and will lower serum potassium levels significantly. These are useful measures in the emergency management of hyperkalemia. Potassium excretion is not affected, so total body potassium will remain elevated.

10. Cation exchange resins such as polystyrene sulfonate lower potassium levels more slowly but are useful because they actually remove potassium from the body. Kayexalate is a sodium cycle exchange resin that exchanges 1.7–2.5 mEq Na^+ for each mEq K^+ that is removed. It must be remembered that Na^+ is added in the exchange; therefore, sodium overload is a potential complication of this therapy.

11. Laboratory studies are used in patients with renal failure to monitor substances that may be abnormal (e.g., Mg^{++}, Ca^{++}, phosphates, creatinine) and to detect factors that may be complicating the condition (e.g., infection). In patients with a sudden or recent onset of renal failure or deterioration, the causes of renal failure that can be treated, including gout, analgesic abuse, infection, obstruction, volume depletion, lupus, and others, must be carefully sought.

12. Special:
Cardiac monitor: chart QRS complex width q 1 h
10% calcium gluconate 10 ml at bedside

12. The ECG in patients with hyperkalemia typically contains tall, peaked T waves, absence of P waves, or a widened QRS complex. In this patient, the width of the QRS complex was a useful sign to monitor the effect of therapy. Calcium can immediately counteract the cardiac toxicity of hyperkalemia, especially if hypocalcemia is present. It should not be given to patients receiving digitalis.

HYPONATREMIA

1. Admit to 5 South

1. Patients are often admitted to an intensive care unit if significant neurologic symptoms are present.

2. Diagnosis: Hyponatremia, probable SIADH, small cell carcinoma of lung

2. Hyponatremia is a common occurrence in hospitalized patients. Patients may be asymptomatic or may experience symptoms ranging from malaise and apathy to confusion, muscle twitching, stupor, seizures, or coma. Hyponatremia is associated with a number of illnesses (including congestive heart failure, cirrhosis, nephrosis, adrenal insufficiency, renal failure, water intoxication, and SIADH [syndrome of inappropriate antidiuretic hormone]) and may also be artifactual in patients with marked hyperglycemia and hyperlipidemia. It was believed that this patient had SIADH related to small cell carcinoma of the lung, and although his lung cancer was relatively stable, he entered the hospital with hyponatremia (serum Na of 118 mEq/L), water excess, and normovolemia. He was somewhat apathetic and confused but otherwise had a normal examination.

3. Condition: Critical

3. Routine.

4. Allergies: NKA

4. Routine.

5. Vital Signs: Temp, BP, Pulse, Resp q 4 h with neurologic checks; postural BP every day
   Call physician if:
   BP < 90 systolic
   Temp > 38.5° C (PO)
   Change in mental status or seizures
   Daily weights

5. Recording vital signs monitors the patient's fluid volume and neurologic status. Treatment should be more aggressive if the patient shows neurologic deterioration.

6. Activity: Bed rest; up in a chair, as tolerated

6. Routine.

7. Nursing:
   Seizure precautions (see "Seizures" under "Neurologic Diseases")
   500 ml fluid restriction (250 ml dietary and 250 ml nursing)
   Strict I and O

7. The nursing staff should monitor the patient's fluid restriction and should be aware of the imminent danger of neurologic deterioration. The nurses may also be asked to maintain a flow chart of blood and urine chemistries, vital signs, and I and O.

8. Diet: House; 250 ml dietary fluid restriction

8. Water restriction is the key element in the treatment of hyponatremia. The restriction is usually divided between nursing and dietary needs. It is important that the patient, nurses, and dietitians understand exactly what the limits are and that they follow them strictly.

9. IV Orders: Heparin lock

9. IV therapy is usually not necessary in the treatment of hyponatremia, except in the rare case of severe hyponatremia (serum Na < 110 mEq/L) or in patients with neurologic complications (stupor, coma, or seizures). If these complications occur, one useful treatment is to administer intravenous furosemide followed by hourly replacement of urinary sodium and potassium losses with 3% hypertonic saline or normal saline (amounts are based on hourly measurements of these losses). Such therapy is usually not required, but if necessary, it can correct hyponatremia enough to eliminate the neurologic symptoms in

6–8 hours. Aggressive treatment of hyponatremia is usually stopped when the serum sodium concentration reaches 120 mEq/L.

10. Medications:
   Routine: DOSS 250 mg PO qd

10. If possible, medications affecting mental status should be avoided. In addition, since most oral drugs must be given with water, a good policy is to minimize the use of any medication in these patients.

11. Laboratory:
   Admission: Simultaneous serum Na and osmolality, urine Na and osmolality; electrolytes, Ca^{++}, glucose, triglycerides, creatinine, BUN, alkaline phosphatase; save serum to observe for lactescence; CBC, CXR (PA and lateral), ECG

11. In SIADH, patients have lost their ability to excrete a water load and thus develop hyponatremia owing to water retention, which is exacerbated by obligatory urinary losses of sodium because of volume expansion. Criteria for diagnosing SIADH are:
   A. Hyponatremia with serum hypo-osmolality.
   B. Inappropriately high urine osmolality, i.e., less than maximally dilute and generally greater than plasma osmolality.
   C. Normal renal, thyroid, and adrenal function.
   D. Inappropriately high urinary sodium.
   E. No evidence of volume depletion or edema. Abnormalities usually disappear following water restriction. In some patients, adrenal function will need to be examined with an ACTH stimulation test and thyroid function will need to be measured with serum TSH level and/or a thyroid screen.

12. Special: None

12. As indicated.

NEPHROLITHIASIS

1. Admit to 5 South

1. Patients are usually admitted to a general medicine or urology service.

2. Diagnosis: Nephrolithiasis

2. Patients with kidney stones are admitted to the hospital primarily for observation and

analgesia. Occasionally, stones must be removed surgically, but usually they pass spontaneously.

3. Condition: Satisfactory

3. Routine.

4. Allergies: NKA

4. Routine.

5. Vital Signs: Temp, BP, Pulse, Resp q.i.d.
   Call physician if:
   Temp > 38.5°C
   BP < 90 systolic
   Daily weights

5. Routine.

6. Activity: Ad lib

6. Routine.

7. Nursing:
   Strain all urine
   I and O

7. The urine is strained in the hope of finding a stone to analyze it.

8. Diet: House; push fluids

8. Patients are often in so much pain that IV hydration is required. They can, however, be offered oral feeding.

9. IV Orders: #1–3. 1000 ml D5–½NS with 20 mEq KCl at 125 ml/h

9. IV fluids are used to correct volume depletion and to maintain a good urine flow. If urate stones are suspected, the patient's urine should be alkalized.

10. Medications:
    Meperidine 100 mg and hydroxyzine 25 mg IM q 2 h prn for pain
    Routine:
    MOM 30 ml PO q hs prn for constipation
    DOSS 250 mg PO qd
    Triazolam 0.25 mg PO q hs prn for sleep

10. The pain of renal colic typically is excruciating. Analgesics should be potent and available at frequent intervals.

11. Laboratory:
    Admission: CBC, SMA-12, uric acid, UA, urine C and S, CXR (PA and lateral); IVP—indication: renal stones (to be done as soon as possible); 24-h urine collection for uric acid, calcium, and creatinine

11. An intravenous pyelogram is used to evaluate the size and location of the stone. Alternatively, ultrasonography can be employed to detect ureteral obstruction and possible resultant hydronephrosis. In addition, patients are evaluated for hypercalciuria or hyperuricosuria. Ideally, the 24-hour urine collection should be done when the patient is on a usual diet (not while NPO!) and may be done after the acute episode has resolved. Those who overpro-

duce uric acid or overexcrete calcium can receive chemoprophylaxis against kidney stone recurrence. Chest x-ray should only be done if indicated.

12. Special: None

12. Urologic consultation is useful, primarily for patients with stones that have not passed.

NEPHROTIC SYNDROME

1. Admit to 5 South

1. Patients are usually admitted to a general medicine floor.

2. Diagnosis: Nephrotic syndrome, hypertension

2. Patients with nephrotic syndrome are often admitted for diagnostic evaluation and management of edema and hypertension.

3. Condition: Satisfactory

3. Routine.

4. Allergies: NKA

4. Routine.

5. Vital Signs: Temp, BP, Pulse, Resp q.i.d.
Call physician if:
BP < 90 or > 180 systolic or > 120 diastolic
Pulse < 55
Temp > 38.5°C
Daily weights

5. Routine.

6. Activity: Bed rest, elevate legs while in bed

6. Elevation will help to mobilize the edema fluid.

7. Nursing:
I and O
Assist with foot care

7. Dermatitis and fissuring can be associated with severe edema. Good foot care is important.

8. Diet: 2 g sodium; 1000 ml fluid restriction

8. Sodium and water intake should be restricted as much as possible in patients with nephrotic syndrome.

9. IV Orders: None

9. Routine

10. Medications:
Furosemide 40 mg PO qd
KCl elixir 20 mEq PO b.i.d.
Propranolol 20 mg PO b.i.d.
Triazolam 0.25 mg PO q hs prn for sleep

10. The mobilization of edema requires the use of diuretics in most cases. Hypertension can be extremely difficult to treat; often beta-blockers and vasodilators in high doses are required. If the patient has renal failure, the drug dosage

and use of KCl should be adjusted accordingly.

11. Laboratory:
Admission: CBC, SMA-12, ANA, cholesterol, TSH, CXR (PA and lateral), ECG, UA, urine C and S, C3, C4 and CH_{50} levels, 24-h urine collection for creatinine and protein

11. The purpose of the laboratory evaluation is to determine the cause of the nephrotic syndrome and the severity of the proteinuria, hypoalbuminemia, and renal failure, if present. Biopsy is not often done in adult nephrotic syndrome, since currently the results of biopsy are not likely to alter the therapy.

12. Special: None

12. As indicated.

RESPIRATORY DISEASES

ASTHMA

1. Admit to the ICU

1. The choice of a medical floor versus the ICU depends on the severity of the illness, the availability of nurses and respiratory therapists, and hospital policy. Some hospitals routinely admit patients in status asthmaticus to the ICU if emergency room (ER) therapy is unsuccessful.

2. Diagnosis: Status asthmaticus

2. Hospitalization for an asthma attack is necessary only if there is severe impairment of the patient's respiratory function that does not show rapid, objective improvement with therapy, which is usually given in the ER. Most patients admitted with asthma will have already received 2–3 hours of therapy, including inhaled and subcutaneous sympathomimetics, oxygen, IV fluids, and perhaps corticosteroids and IV methylxanthines. In spite of therapy, these patients do not show improvement in peak expiratory flow, FEV_1, arterial oxygen level, or some other easily measured parameter. In addition, they usually remain uncomfortable and may be exhausted from their increased respiratory workload.

3. Condition: Critical

3. Most patients admitted to the ICU are in critical condition.

4. Allergies: NKA; avoid ASA-containing medications

4. Approximately 10% of patients with asthma are sensitive to aspirin; these patients also may react to tartrazine, yellow dye No. 5, indomethacin, other nonsteroidal antiinflammatory drugs (NSAIDs), and aminopyrine.

5. Vital Signs: ICU routine q 1 h
   Measure and chart pulsus paradoxus
   Call physician if:
     Resp < 12 or > 30
     Pulse > 130

5. Taking vital signs monitors the patient for impending respiratory failure (rapid respiratory rate or slow rate, if exhausted; rapid heart rate; increasing pulsus paradoxus; and altered consciousness).

Xanthine or sympathomimetic toxicity may be reflected in persistent tachycardia (heart rate > 130).

6. Activity: Bed rest; may use commode and sit in a chair, if able

6. Patients should be allowed to rest in the position that is most comfortable for them. Most prefer to sit.

7. Nursing:
   I and O
   Daily weights
   Measure bedside peak expiratory flow q 2 h with portable peak flowmeter
   Record vital signs, pulsus paradoxus, ABGs, VC, FEV_1, and peak expiratory flow (before and after isoetharine) on flow chart

7. The nursing staff should make frequent observations to determine the patient's response to therapy and to assess the need for intubation and mechanical ventilation. They can also measure bronchospasm (using a peak flowmeter) before and after therapy with inhaled bronchodilators to determine its effectiveness (some patients may actually have increased bronchospasm after inhaling bronchodilators). FEV_1 (forced expiratory volume in one second), as measured by bedside spirometry, can also be used to follow a patient's progress.

8. Diet: House, when tolerated

8. In status asthmaticus, most patients will not want to eat, and if intubation seems likely, they should remain NPO. However, as soon as patients improve or have an appetite and are not likely to require intubation they should eat a normal diet.

9. IV Orders:
   #1. 1000 ml D5–½NS and 20 mEq KCl at 175 ml/h
   #2. 1000 ml D5–½NS and 20 mEq KCl at 125 ml/h
   #3. 1000 ml D5–½NS and 20 mEq KCl at 125 ml/h

9. Fluid intake should be high (3000–3500 ml/day) to maintain adequate hydration and to ensure that secretions continue to be loosened. Patients receiving corticosteroids commonly develop hypokalemia. In addition, patients with acute respiratory failure usually secrete excess ADH and are prone to develop hyponatremia if excessive free water is administered.

10. Medications:
    Methylprednisolone 125 mg IV q 6 h
    Albuterol 3 mg in 2.5 ml NS via nebulizer q 4 h for 24 h

10. Most patients admitted with status asthmaticus should receive corticosteroids, although the dosage is a matter of controversy. Methylpred-

Routine: None
NO SEDATIVES

nisolone 1–2 mg/kg IV q 6 h is a standard dose, administered for 48 hours and then tapered. Lower doses of corticosteroids are usually also effective. Some authorities recommend much higher doses (e.g., 1 g methylprednisolone q 6 h) calculated according to the severity of the patient's bronchospasm.

Sympathomimetics are receiving increasing recognition for their important role in treating bronchospasm. Most patients will receive subcutaneous epinephrine or terbutaline in the ER, and virtually every patient should receive inhaled beta-agonists on a regular schedule during an acute exacerbation.

Methylxanthines are currently reserved for the treatment of acute asthma in patients who fail to improve on maximal inhaled bronchodilator therapy (e.g., albuterol). Methylxanthines are potentially useful as both bronchodilator and stimulant for fatigued respiratory muscles. If employed, a loading dose of aminophylline, 4–6 mg/kg over 15–30 min is usually required in patients who are not receiving routine outpatient theophylline. The maintenance dose is more difficult to calculate and is subject to extreme variations in metabolic degradation in different patients under different curcumstances, but it is usually in the range of 0.3–0.9 mg/kg/h. When intravenous aminophylline is being administered, serum theophylline levels should be followed to guide dosing. Therapeutic concentrations are greater than 10 μg/ml. The frequency of side effects increases with levels greater than 20 μg/ml. Toxicity includes anxiety, agitation, and cardiac arrhythmias. Use of infusion pumps can help prevent problems due to fluctuating blood levels and minimize the chance of accidental overdose from inadvertent rapid infusion.

11. Laboratory:
    Admission: CBC, SMA-12, CXR, ECG, ABGs, sputum Gram stain and culture, UA (already done in ER)
    Repeat ABGs in 6 h
    Tomorrow: Hct, WBC, electrolytes, ABGs

11. Patients should be evaluated for the presence of infection (Gram stain, chest x-ray) and for evidence of electrolyte imbalance and dehydration. Monitoring the ABGs is helpful in the assessment of the patient's clinical course. Other diagnoses to consider include airway obstruction due to a foreign body, tumor, pulmonary embolus, pulmonary edema, exacerbation of chronic bronchitis, and anaphylaxis.

12. Special:
    Respiratory therapist to see patient q shift and as needed for first 24 h
    1. Chest physiotherapy (PT) and postural drainage, if tolerated and if helpful in raising secretions, thereby improving FEV_1
    2. Measure VC and FEV_1 q shift
    3. O_2 at 2 L/min by nasal prongs

12. Contrary to traditional beliefs, use of IPPB is not helpful in asthma and may even increase bronchospasm. Respiratory therapy with chest PT and postural drainage may be helpful for patients with infiltrates and for those who find it difficult to raise secretions. The therapists can also assist in monitoring respiratory function.

CHRONIC OBSTRUCTIVE PULMONARY DISEASE (COPD) AND BRONCHITIS

1. Admit to 5 South

1. Patients with COPD can usually be admitted to a general medicine floor.

2. Diagnosis: Chronic bronchitis with emphysema and superimposed acute bronchitis

2. The exacerbation of underlying respiratory insufficiency by an acute infection (bronchitis or pneumonia) is the most common reason for admitting a patient with COPD to the hospital. The infection may also precipitate increased bronchospasm and lead to volume depletion.

3. Condition: Serious

3. Routine.

4. Allergies: NKA

4. Routine.

5. Vital Signs: BP, Pulse, Resp, Temp q 4 h
   Call physician if:
   Temp > 38.5°C
   BP < 90 systolic
   Resp < 12 or > 30
   Pulse > 130
   Daily weights

5. Taking vital signs monitors the patient for evidence of respiratory failure, volume depletion, and progressive infection.

6. Activity: Ad lib in room

6. Routine.

7. Nursing:
   Measure peak flow with portable peak flowmeter b.i.d. and chart with vital signs
   I and O

7. A portable peak flowmeter can be used to assess the patient's response to therapy. It can also be used to measure airway resistance before and after chest physiotherapy.

8. Diet: No added salt; push fluids

8. Patients with right heart failure may require more stringent salt restriction.

9. IV Orders:
   Heparin lock–rt. arm

9. Routine.

10. Medications: Ampicillin 1 g IV q 6 H
    Albuterol 3 mg in 2.5 ml NS q 4 h by nebulizer
    Routine: DOSS 250 mg PO q AM
    NO SEDATIVES

10. This patient's Gram stain showed leukocytes and a predominance of gram-negative coccobacillary organisms, suggesting infection with *Hemophilus influenzae*. Ampicillin is the treatment of choice and was given IV, although the oral route would also have been adequate. Inhaled bronchodilators help to improve the bronchospasm associated with chronic bronchitis and allow for easier clearance of secretions. As in the treatment of asthma, sedatives are to be avoided, since they can suppress the patient's respiratory drive and cough reflex, thereby contributing to respiratory failure.

    Selected patients with chronic bronchitis benefit from methylxanthine bronchodilators. However, inhaled sympathomimetic amines (e.g., albuterol) are the drug(s) of choice for therapeutic bronchodilation in the management of COPD. When added to a regimen of inhaled sympathomimetic bronchodilator, methylxanthines often contribute only to toxicity (e.g., tachycardia, arrhythmias, anxiety) rather than to therapeutic efficacy. Therefore, methylxanthines should be reserved for patients in whom intensive inhaled sympathomimetic therapy fails. If used, aminophylline should be first administered as a loading dose (5 mg/kg IV). The patient on chronic therapy does not necessarily require a loading dose, and the maintenance dose is usually 0.3–0.9 mg/kg/h. The doses are reduced in the presence of hepatic, renal, or cardiac insufficiency. Oral therapy may be adequate in some cases. Good hydration will promote expectoration.

11. Laboratory:
    Admission: CBC, ABGs, electrolytes, BUN, glucose, UA, CXR (done), sputum for Gram stain and culture, ECG (done)
    Tomorrow: ABGs

11. The Gram stain of expectorated sputum should be examined in all patients for the presence of infection and to help in the selection of antibiotics. Other laboratory studies assess the severity of hypoxemia and hypercarbia and reveal electrolyte abnormalities. Determination of a theophylline level may be helpful in some patients.

12. Special:
    Continuous O_2 at 2 L/min with nebulized air by nasal prongs
    Respiratory therapist to assist patient with postural drainage and chest wall percussion

12. High-flow oxygen may suppress the respiratory drive in patients with chronic hypercarbia and should be avoided. However, low-flow oxygen can be used to improve hypoxemia. Such therapy reduces pulmonary hypertension and makes patients more responsive to pharmacotherapy and more comfortable.
    The respiratory therapist can help patients to expectorate secretions. In addition, patients may be taught techniques that they can use at home.

HEMOPTYSIS WITH LUNG MASS

1. Admit to 5 North

1. Most patients with hemoptysis can be observed on a gen-

eral medicine ward. Occasionally, a patient will have massive hemoptysis and need urgent surgery. If an underlying pulmonary disease is severe enough (as in many cigarette smokers), admission to an ICU may be appropriate.

If tuberculosis is suspected, a ward with respiratory isolation is necessary.

2. Diagnosis: Hemoptysis, lung mass

2. Most cases of hemoptysis are minor and occur with episodes of bronchitis or other infections. In the setting of a lung mass, the likelihood of a carcinoma is increased, particularly in patients with a history of smoking. Occasionally pneumonia, lung abscess, tuberculosis, or Wegener's granulomatosis can present with hemoptysis associated with a mass lesion on chest x-ray. A careful history and physical examination are the two most important parts of the evaluation and will help establish a reasonable provisional diagnosis in most cases.

3. Condition: Serious

3. The potential always exists for massive hemoptysis, particularly with necrotic infections or other lesions that could erode larger blood vessels.

4. Allergies: NKA

4. Routine.

5. Vital Signs: BP, Pulse, Temp, Resp q.i.d. when awake
   Call physician if:
   BP > 140 or < 100 systolic
   Temp > 38°C
   Pulse > 140 or < 60
   Resp > 25 or < 10

5. Routine monitoring of vital signs is adequate unless hemoptysis is massive. An increase in respiration rate may indicate occult bleeding.

6. Activity: Bed rest, bedside commode privileges

6. During the first 48 hours patients should be carefully watched, as recurrent, massive bleeding may occur without warning.

7. Nursing:
   Collect all sputum and expectorated blood in a bedside container

7. Quantitation of hemoptysis may provide prognostic information, as the patient's estimate is frequently not accu-

I and O
Daily weights

8. Diet: NPO × 24 h, then clear liquids

9. IV Orders:
   #1. 1000 ml D5–½NS + 20 mEq KCl × 100 ml/h
   #2. 1000 ml D5–½NS + 20 mEq KCl × 100 ml/h
   #3. IV to heparin lock until further notice

10. Medications:
    Ampicillin 500 mg IV q 6 h
    Codeine 30 mg PO q 6 h

11. Laboratory:
    Admission: CBC, SMA-12, PT, PTT, CXR (done); ECG, ABG; sputum for Gram stain and culture, for AFB, q AM × 3, and for cytology q AM × 3
    Tomorrow AM: Repeat CXR

12. Special:
    Thoracic surgery consult
    Pulmonary consult

rate. Blood loss greater than 600 ml in less than 48 hours constitutes an emergency and necessitates a rigid bronchoscopy and consideration of surgery.

8. Until the magnitude of bleeding is determined, patients should be considered as preoperative patients and thus maintained on an empty stomach.

9. Maintenance fluids are necessary since the patient is not receiving oral intake. When fluids are discontinued, a heparin lock should be maintained for several days in case there is a need for emergency evaluation or for treatment of recurrent bleeding.

10. Treatment of infection is important, particularly if patients have purulent sputum or evidence of bronchitis. Bronchospasm may occur and should be treated accordingly but is usually a problem only with more severe chronic lung disease. Because coughing may precipitate further hemoptysis, codeine is administered as an antitussive, but dosages should be held for somnolence.

11. If the bleeding subsides, results of both AFB and cytologic studies may help direct therapy. Sputum cytology is the preferred diagnostic method for detecting small cell carcinoma but is less helpful for other malignancies. Special precautions must be taken in AFB-positive patients. A repeat CXR in the morning may help judge the status of bleeding.

12. Both thoracic surgery and pulmonary consultants should be aware of the patient. If hemoptysis is minor, and if sputum cytology and other diagnostic studies are not

conclusive, the patient will probably need fiberoptic bronchoscopy for both a diagnosis and staging. Thoracic surgeons may be needed for rigid bronchoscopy or for operative intervention.

PNEUMONIA

(See Sample orders in Part I, Section 2, "Components of Admitting Orders.")

RESPIRATORY FAILURE

1. Admit to the ICU

1. Routine.

2. Diagnosis: Respiratory failure, viral pneumonia, influenza

2. Respiratory failure is defined as a failure of the respiratory system to provide for an exchange of oxygen and carbon dioxide between the environment and the body tissues in quantities sufficient to sustain life. The cause of this failure can be located in the brain (e.g., drug overdose), spinal cord and muscles (e.g., myasthenia gravis), chest wall (e.g., flail chest), upper airways (e.g., laryngospasm or edema), lower airways and lungs (e.g., asthma, ARDS, pneumonias), or heart (e.g., pulmonary edema). By general standards, respiratory failure is present when the arterial $pO_2 < 50$ mm Hg; the arterial $pCO_2 > 60$ (except in chronic hypercapnea); the respiratory rate is > 35; the inspiratory force is < 25 cm H_2O; or the vital capacity is < 15 ml/kg. Intubation and mechanical ventilation are usually indicated when patients develop such severe respiratory failure. The care of these critically ill patients must be individualized, and only general guidelines will be presented here.

3. Condition: Critical

3. Routine.

4. Allergies: NKA

4. Often, allergies cannot be determined in these patients.

5. Vital Signs: ICU routine q 1 h, including ECG monitor and arterial pressure tracing from arterial line

5. Careful monitoring of the vital signs of these extremely ill patients will usually be done by ICU protocol and is of utmost importance. An arterial line also makes it easier to obtain frequent ABGs.

6. Activity: Bed rest

6. Routine.

7. Nursing:
I and O
Daily weights
NG tube
Foley catheter
Maintain flow chart with all vital signs, electrolytes, ABGs, ventilator settings, and lung compliance

7. Well-organized flow charts permit the physicians and nurses to accurately follow the patient's clinical course. Without such a careful compilation of data, clinicians are often overwhelmed by masses of disorganized information.

8. Diet: NPO

8. Routine.

9. IV Orders:
#1–3. 1000 ml D5–¼NS with 20 mEq KCl at 100 ml/h for next 24 h

9. IV fluids will replace existing volume deficits and expected losses and correct electrolyte imbalances. Swan-Ganz catheterization or other hemodynamic monitoring is often required to assess the patient's volume status.

10. Medications:
Morphine 1–3 mg IV q 1–2 h prn for sedation
Pancuronium bromide 5 mg IV before intubation, then 1–2 mg IV prn for control of respiratory rate and paralysis
Sucralfate 1 g per NG q 6 h

10. Patients receiving controlled ventilation, especially those with stiff lungs, usually require respiratory paralysis to restrain rapid, inefficient respiratory rates. Sedation is also important, both to control rapid respiratory rates and especially to relieve the terror most patients experience when paralyzed. Sucralfate helps to prevent GI bleeding from stress ulcers.

11. Laboratory:
Admission: CBC, ABGs, SMA-12, CXR, ECG, UA, blood cultures × 2, sputum culture (viral and bacterial), and Gram stain (already done)
Portable CXR immediately after intubation
ABGs 30 min after intubation, then at least qd
Electrolytes and hematocrit qd

11. A chest x-ray is essential to assess tube placement, and ABGs will determine the ventilator settings. Otherwise, laboratory studies are used to guide oxygen concentration and electrolyte and fluid therapy and, eventually, to document the patient's response to therapy.

12. Special:

Anesthesia to intubate patient as soon as possible (called)

Ventilator settings:

MA–1 initial settings;

Tidal volume—800 ml

PEEP—0

Rate—12/min

FiO_2—100% until ABGs are drawn, then decrease to 50%

Call physician for further settings as soon as postintubation ABGs are available

Arterial line: Routine care

NG tube: Routine care

Airway care per nursing and respiratory therapy protocol

12. An elective intubation by an anesthesiologist is preferable to a poorly planned emergency intubation. The settings of the ventilator depend on the ventilations per minute required to ensure an adequate alveolar ventilation as determined by arterial blood gases. A tidal volume of 10–12 ml/kg and a rate of 10–12/min are usually reasonable starting points. The FiO_2 is adjusted to maintain the PaO_2 above 60 mm Hg, which will usually give at least a 90% O_2 saturation. Little is gained by striving for a PaO_2 higher than the 60s. Furthermore, oxygen toxicity and airway trauma from overly vigorous use of PEEP can be minimized by not aiming for higher PaO_2 levels. Orders for ventilator patients are also described in detail on pages 182–183 in the section "Orders Accompanying Procedures."

RHEUMATIC DISEASES

GOUT

1. Admit to 5 North

1. Patients are usually admitted to a general medicine floor.

2. Diagnosis: Gout, podagra—lt. foot

2. Most patients with acute gout attacks are managed as outpatients. However, an occasional patient requires admission for bed rest, medication supervision, or for such severe pain that inpatient management is advisable.

3. Condition: Satisfactory

3. Routine.

4. Allergies: NKA

4. Routine.

5. Vital Signs: BP, Pulse, Temp, Resp q.i.d.
   Call physician if:
   Temp > 38.5°C
   BP < 90 systolic

5. Fever can occur with an acute attack of gout. Nevertheless, the possibility of a coexistent infection causing the fever should be evaluated.

6. Activity: Bed rest; elevate lt. foot until attack subsides

6. Elevation of the affected part reduces edema, thereby decreasing pain.

7. Nursing:
   Support bed sheets with a frame so they do not touch inflamed area of foot

7. Acute gout causes severe pain with edema, erythema, and exquisite sensitivity to touch. Therefore, elevation and supports designed to prevent contact with the inflamed area are helpful.

8. Diet: No added salt

8. Routine.

9. IV Orders: None

9. Occasionally, patients with gout will have severe nausea, vomiting, or volume depletion and will require IV fluids.

10. Medications:
    Indomethacin 50 mg PO q.i.d. with food
    Ranitidine 150 mg PO b.i.d.
    Routine:
    DOSS 250 mg PO qd
    MOM 30 ml PO q hs prn for constipation
    Triazolam 0.25 mg PO q hs prn for sleep

10. Because they have fewer side effects, nonsteroidal antiinflammatory agents such as indomethacin, naproxen, sulindac, and other NSAIDs have replaced colchicine as the treatment of choice for acute gout. Colchicine may be helpful diagnostically or can be given IV to patients who cannot take oral medications. High doses of NSAIDs are usually given for 24 hours only and then tapered over 3–5 days.
    Not all patients require urate-lowering drug therapy (e.g., allopurinol, probenecid,

sulfinpyrazone). Urate-lowering therapy is usually reserved for patients with recurrent attacks. However, this type of therapy should not be initiated until the gout attack subsides. Patients who are beginning treatment with urate-lowering medications should be covered with prophylactic colchicine (0.6 mg b.i.d.) during the initial phase of therapy to prevent flare-ups of gout.

11. Laboratory:
    Admission: CBC with differential, SMA-12, uric acid, UA, CXR (PA and lateral), ECG; send joint fluid for C and S, cell count, Gram stain (micrography for crystals and Gram stain have been performed, in addition); 24-h urine for uric acid, creatinine

11. In addition to the routine admission laboratory work, one of the most important studies is microscopic examination of the joint fluid for crystals using a polarizing filter and, if available, a red lens. The observation of thin, negatively birefringent crystals in the neutrophils is diagnostic of gout. Cultures of the joint fluid are used to evaluate the possibility of infection, and a 24-hour urine for determination of uric acid excretion and uric acid level will allow patients to be classified as overproducers or underexcretors.

12. Special: None

12. As indicated.

RHEUMATOID ARTHRITIS

1. Admit to 5 North

1. Patients are usually admitted to a general medicine floor.

2. Diagnosis: Rheumatoid arthritis, active

2. Patients with rheumatoid arthritis are admitted for diagnosis, surgery, and in-hospital therapy of disease flare-ups and complications such as infections (see "Septic Arthritis" pp. 101–104) and GI bleeding. This patient was admitted for in-hospital therapy of active disease.

3. Condition: Satisfactory

3. Routine.

4. Allergies: NKA

4. Routine.

5. Vital Signs: Temp, BP, Pulse, Resp t.i.d.

5. Routine.

Call physician if:
Temp > 38.5°C
BP < 90 systolic

6. Activity: Bed rest with bathroom privileges

6. Bed rest is an important adjunct to medication and physical therapy for patients with active rheumatoid arthritis. In some instances, admission to the hospital may be necessary simply to assure that the patient has sufficient bed rest.

7. Nursing:
Patient is to use resting wrist splints as much as possible.

7. The nursing staff can help the patient to use the appliances and splints provided by the physical therapist. They may also help to perform physical therapy.

8. Diet: House

8. Routine.

9. IV Orders: None

9. Routine.

10. Medications:
Aspirin 900 mg PO q 4 h when awake, 1200 mg PO q hs
Prednisone 15 mg PO qd
Ranitidine 150 mg PO b.i.d.
Routine:
DOSS 250 mg PO qd
MOM 30 ml PO q hs prn for constipation
Triazolam 0.25 mg PO q hs prn for sleep; may repeat once

10. Drug therapy for patients with rheumatoid arthritis must be individualized. Salicylates have traditionally been the foundation of all drug therapy. Increasingly, however, newer NSAIDs, such as naproxen, sulindac, and ibuprofen, are being used in lieu of aspirin. Steroids may be administered to help control acute inflammation, but they should be given at the lowest effective dose and not at all if remission can be obtained using agents such as gold, penicillamine, or methotrexate. However, the goals of therapy are to minimize the acute inflammation and then to develop a program to induce a remission. Many clinicians prefer to administer chronic antiulcer prophylaxis to patients maintained on long-term aspirin, corticosteroid, or NSAID therapy to reduce the risk of gastrointestinal bleeding. Ranitidine 150 mg PO b.i.d., sucralfate 1 g PO q.i.d. (1 h before each meal and q hs), or misoprostol 200 μg PO q.i.d. is a reasonable regimen.

11. Laboratory:
    Admission: CBC, ESR, SMA-12, rheumatoid factor, ANA, UA, CXR (PA and lateral), hand x-rays, ECG

11. Most patients with previously diagnosed rheumatoid arthritis do not require extensive laboratory evaluations. The titer of the rheumatoid factor (latex fixation) has prognostic significance in that patients with high titers do not fare as well (especially if they have nodules).

12. Special:
    Physical therapist to see patient for evaluation and PT at least every day
    Jacuzzi baths, if possible, q AM
    Bilateral resting wrist splints

12. Physical therapy is an extremely important part of the treatment for those with active rheumatoid arthritis, and patients can be taught management techniques that they can use at home. Warm baths provide much symptomatic relief of joint discomfort and stiffness.

SYSTEMIC LUPUS ERYTHEMATOSUS (SLE)

1. Admit to 5 South

1. Patients are usually admitted to a general medicine floor.

2. Diagnosis: Systemic lupus erythematosus, pleuropericarditis, fever

2. Patients with lupus are admitted to manage flare-ups of the disease and complications of therapy and for diagnostic evaluation. This patient had a recurrence of pleuropericarditis, a common manifestation of the polyserositis seen in patients with SLE.

3. Condition: Satisfactory

3. Routine.

4. Allergies: NKA

4. Routine.

5. Vital Signs: Temp, BP, Pulse, Resp q 4 h; take and chart pulsus paradoxus with BP
    Call physician if:
    BP < 90 systolic
    Resp > 25
    Pulsus paradoxus > 25
    Pulse pressure < 15

5. Although cardiac tamponade is extremely rare in lupus pericarditis, the patient's vital signs, including level of pulsus paradoxus, are monitored to detect its occurrence.

6. Activity: Bed rest with bathroom privileges

6. Bed rest is a time-honored treatment of acute flare-ups in most rheumatic diseases.

7. Nursing:
    Flow charts should include level of pulsus paradoxus

7. Flow charts are a helpful means of organizing clinical data.

8. Diet: No added salt

8. Routine.

9. IV Orders: None

9. Routine.

10. Medications:
    Prednisone 20 mg PO t.i.d.
    Ranitidine 150 mg PO b.i.d.
    Routine:
    MOM 30 ml PO q hs prn for
    constipation
    Triazolam 0.25 mg PO q hs
    prn for sleep
    Acetaminophen 650 mg PO q
    4 h prn for pain

10. Corticosteroids are the cornerstone of drug therapy for patients with SLE who do not respond to salicylates and nonsteroidal anti-inflammatory drugs. The dose to be given depends on the severity of the patient's condition, past responses to steroids, and the dose regimen at the time of disease flare-up.

11. Laboratory:
    Admission: CBC, ESR, SMA-12, UA, CXR (PA and lateral), ECG, DNA-binding, urine culture, blood cultures × 2, sputum culture (if available)
    Repeat CXR (PA and lateral) in 3 days—indication: follow-up of pleural and pericardial effusions

11. In patients who are known to have lupus, the clinical response to therapy as well as the laboratory parameters of disease activity are followed. Many of the latter exist, and all need not be followed routinely. In this patient, the level of antibody to double-stranded DNA (DNA-binding), CBC, and ESR are the pertinent laboratory studies. Patients with SLE should be evaluated for possible infection, which can cause flare-ups of the disease and fever.

12. Special: Echocardiogram—indication: to evaluate pericardial effusion and rule out cardiac tamponade physiology (schedule as soon as possible).

12. An echocardiogram should be obtained to evaluate the size of the pericardial effusion. The presence of cardiac tamponade (e.g., diastolic inversion of the ventricular wall) demands urgent cardiology consultation and consideration of pericardiocentesis.

PART III

ORDERS ACCOMPANYING PROCEDURES

ARTERIAL LINE

Arterial lines are used to monitor blood pressure in shock from any cause and during administration of intravenous afterload therapy. Some physicians recommend the use of arterial lines in pulmonary edema and acute respiratory failure. An Allen test should be performed prior to use of the radial artery and the line should be inserted with attention to strict sterile technique. If possible, the line should be removed and changed after 72 hours, as the risk of infection greatly increases if it is left in longer. The patient should be in an intensive care unit, and the distal arterial bed should be monitored closely for any signs of ischemia.

The following orders are indicated after the insertion of an arterial monitoring line:

1. Local care: Cover the area daily with sterile dressings, using neomycin ointment at the entry site.

2. Heparin flush (2 ml of heparin per 500 ml D5W): Place on a continuous infusion system of 3 ml/h.

3. Place an armboard with a roll under the wrist for hyperextension of the wrist.

ASPIRATION CATHETER FOR TREATMENT OF PNEUMOTHORAX

Small-bore percutaneous aspiration catheters are now the method of choice to treat pneumothorax. They do not require an incision and avoid many of the problems associated with large-bore chest tubes. With some spontaneous pneumothoraces in young patients, the catheter is attached to a Heimlich valve and taped to the chest wall, and the patient's progress is followed on an outpatient basis after the patient's discharge from the hospital.

PRE-CATHETERIZATION

1. Diet: NPO

2. Scrub anterior chest wall

3. Aspiration catheter at bedside

4. Heimlich valve available at bedside

1. Generally, Heimlich valves are used to vent the catheter and to occlude the catheter during inspiration. On occasion, the catheter may be attached to water seal but only rarely to suction.

POST-CATHETERIZATION

1. Portable AP CXR

2. Vital Signs: q 15 min × 4, then q 4 h (BP, Pulse, Resp)

3. Routine dressing changes

4. Call physician for increased respiratory distress

1. Catheter placement must be confirmed by an x-ray. Vital signs should be monitored to ascertain that the patient's condition is stable. In general, patients are admitted to the hospital; some may be discharged if their condition is stable with the catheter in place. Catheters are usually removed in a day or two.

BRONCHOSCOPY

Bronchoscopy is performed to visualize the bronchial tree, collect specimens for culture and pathologic examination, and relieve obstruction. The procedure involves some risk related to the patient's cardiopulmonary status. Complications include arrhythmias, aspiration, and bleeding.

PRE-BRONCHOSCOPY ORDERS

1. Diet: NPO after midnight

1. By making the patient NPO, the risk of aspiration is minimized.

2. Premedication: Atropine 0.8 mg SC 30 min before procedure

2. Premedication preferences vary widely. Atropine is used to minimize proximal bronchospasm and prevent vagally induced arrhythmias. Other drugs used for premedication include midazolam, hydroxyzine, and morphine, or no premedications are given at all.

3. Laboratory: Prothrombin time, platelet count, Hct

3. Laboratory studies assess a patient for bleeding tendencies.

POST-BRONCHOSCOPY ORDERS

1. Vital Signs: Pulse, BP, Resp q 1 h × 2

2. Diet: NPO for 2 h, then try sips of water; if swallowed without difficulty, may resume diet and PO fluids

2. Since the pharynx and proximal airway are anesthetized, before allowing PO fluids the physician must be certain that sensation has returned and that the patient will not aspirate.

3. Laboratory: Post-procedure chest x-ray—indication: Post-bronchoscopy with biopsy.

3. A chest x-ray is taken to detect pneumothorax or aspiration.

CARDIAC CATHETERIZATION

PRE-CARDIAC CATHETERIZATION ORDERS

1. Nursing: Obtain consent for procedure. Prepare the groin (or arm), and have patient void before procedure

1. Routine.

2. Diet: NPO after midnight except usual medications

2. If the procedure is scheduled in the afternoon, the patient can have a clear liquid breakfast.

3. Premedication: Lorazepam 2 mg PO 30 min before procedure

3. Some physicians prefer to use meperidine, 75 mg, and promethazine, 25 mg IM, for pre-procedure sedation. Midazolam can also be useful.

4. IV: Heparin lock

4. Routine.

POST-CARDIAC CATHETERIZATION ORDERS

1. Vital Signs: BP, heart rate, and distal pulse q 30 min × 2, then q 60 min × 2, then q 4 h × 24 h if condition is stable
   Call physician if:
   BP < 100 systolic
   Pulse > 120

1. Changes in the patient's vital signs may indicate blood loss and the development of shock.

2. Activity: Strict bed rest for 6 h, with leg straight at groin; may elevate head of bed 30°

2. The major complications of the postcatheterization period are bleeding and arterial obstruction. Restriction of activity and careful positioning minimize the chance that these complications will occur.

3. Nursing:
   Observe the patient carefully for bleeding at puncture (or cut-down) site and for loss of distal pulse; if bleeding occurs, apply enough direct pressure to stop bleeding but not obliterate the distal pulse; may apply 5-lb sandbag to assist in control of bleeding
   Call physician if bleeding occurs or if patient complains of severe groin pain or angina
   Assist patient with ambulation after 6 h

3. As noted, nursing measures are directed toward controlling any bleeding without causing arterial insufficiency. Early detection of the loss of a pulse is extremely important, since arterial obstruction usually demands urgent intervention.

4. Diet: Encourage fluid intake, 100–200 ml/h

4. Routine.

5. Medications: Acetaminophen 325 mg and codeine 30 mg, 1 or 2 tabs PO q 3 h for pain
   Resume previous diet and medications

5. Routine.

CHEST TUBE PLACEMENT

Chest tubes are placed for traumatic hemothorax or for drainage of the pleural space when simple aspiration is inadequate (for instance, in empyema or malignant effusion). The use of a chest tube is rarely necessary in the nontraumatic setting for treatment of pneumothorax, although this is the pattern of use in many institutions. The use of a chest tube carries a risk of infection as well as other intrathoracic complications. Tubes smaller than 30 French should not be used because of kinking and clotting problems.

PRE-CHEST TUBE PLACEMENT

1. Diet: NPO

   1. Routine.

2. Scrub right chest wall with Betadine

   2. The major complications related to the use of chest tubes are improper placement and secondary infection. The site should be sterile and adequate anesthesia should be assured.

3. Have chest tube tray available at bedside

   3. Routine.

4. Have 2% lidocaine and 30 French catheter at bedside

   4. May vary according to situation.

POST-CHEST TUBE PLACEMENT

1. Connect to 15 cm H_2O suction

   1. Routine.

2. Portable AP and lateral CXR

   2. Lateral chest x-ray is mandatory to determine if tube placement is correct. If placement is incorrect, the tube must be readjusted within an hour, or a separate entry site should be used.

3. Vital Signs: q 15 min × 4, q 1 h × 4, then q 4 h (BP, Pulse, Resp)

   3. Hypotension or severe hypoxemia occasionally occurs after rapid evacuation of the pleural space.

4. Standard dressing changes q d

   4. Routine.

5. Call physician for:
   Erythema or draining at tube site
   Fever > 38°C
   Subcutaneous emphysema

   5. The chest tube should be removed as soon as possible.

ENDOSCOPIC EXAMINATION OF THE COLON

The entire colon can be visualized with colonoscopy. This procedure may be performed for diagnosis (e.g., malignancy, inflammatory bowel disease, polyps) or for biopsies and polypectomies. Colonoscopy is usually done on an outpatient basis.

PRE-COLONOSCOPY ORDERS

1. Nursing: Tap water enemas × 2, PM before procedure; tap water enemas until clear, beginning 3 h before procedure (usually 3–6 enemas)

2. Diet: Only clear liquids for two days prior to procedure; NPO after midnight before procedure

3. Medications: Magnesium citrate 300 mg PO PM before procedure

4. Laboratory: Hct, platelet count, and PT

1–3. The colon must be as clean as possible for the colonoscopy to be effective. Cathartics should be omitted in patients with inflammatory bowel disease if they already have diarrhea or active disease. Enemas, especially in patients with ulcerative colitis, should be given gently.

4. If a biopsy or polypectomy is not anticipated, the patient need not be screened for bleeding tendencies. Patients should also have had a recent ECG. If a biopsy is anticipated, those with valvular heart disease should receive prophylactic treatment for bacterial endocarditis.

POST-COLONOSCOPY ORDERS

1. Nursing: Observe for unusual abdominal, shoulder, or rectal pain or fever; call physician if present

1. Since colonoscopy is commonly performed on an outpatient basis, the patient does not need special monitoring by the nurse, unless complications occurred during the procedure or are anticipated.

ENDOSCOPY OF THE UPPER GI TRACT AND ENDOSCOPIC RETROGRADE CHOLANGIOPANCREATOGRAPHY (ERCP)

Upper gastrointestinal endoscopy allows a direct visualization of the upper GI tract into the duodenum and permits the diagnosis of such diverse conditions as esophagitis, gastritis, ulcers, varices, and malignancies. It can be especially helpful in patients who are bleeding. ERCP involves cannulation of the common duct by endoscopy, injection of contrast media into the pancreatobiliary tree, and x-ray filming. Both procedures are commonly performed on an outpatient basis.

PRE-ENDOSCOPY ORDERS

1. Diet: NPO after midnight

2. Premedications:
   Lorazepam 1 mg IV—on call
   Atropine 0.8 mg IV—on call

3. Laboratory: Platelet count, Hct, and PT

1. Routine.

2. The use of premedication varies according to the patient and the physician. Lorazepam provides sedation and amnesia, and atropine may prevent arrhythmias due to the vagal discharges associated with these procedures.

3. Laboratory studies are indicated in patients who are likely to have a biopsy; otherwise, they need not be ordered routinely.

POST-ENDOSCOPY ORDERS

1. Vital Signs: BP, Pulse, Temp q 2 h × 4, then q 4 h until tomorrow
   Call physician if:
   Temp > 38.0°C
   BP < 90 systolic
   Neck or chest pain, dysphasia, or bleeding

2. Diet: NPO for 2 h, then give patient sips of water; if swallowed without difficulty, resume diet and medications

1. Taking vital signs monitors the patient for evidence of aspiration, perforation, or bleeding.

2. Because the upper airway is anesthetized, eating must be delayed until the patient can swallow without danger of aspirating.

FEEDING TUBE PLACEMENT

Following placement of a nasogastric feeding tube, a CXR should be obtained to verify tube position prior to its use for the administration of medications or nutritional formulas. The radio-opaque tip of a properly placed feeding tube should be in the body of the stomach below the diaphragm.

HICKMAN AND HICKMAN-BROVIAC CATHETER CARE

INSERTION

Procedure done under local anesthesia without need for specific pre-op orders.

ROUTINE CARE

1. Change dressing once daily using sterile technique. Observe exit wound for inflammation or discharge. Apply small amount of Betadine or Neosporin ointment to exit site before redressing. Aspirate line, then flush with 5 ml injectable saline, then instill 3 ml heparin flush solution (100 units/ml) and cap the line

1. Most nursing units have routine procedures for Hickman catheter care.

If unable to aspirate or flush catheter, perform the following steps sequentially:

1. Attempt "rocking" (back and forth) aspiration, and flush using small amount of sterile saline

1. Occasionally, a small thrombus will be aspirated, thus clearing the catheter, or the catheter tip will be dislodged from its position against the vascular wall.

2. Instill 2.5 ml heparin solution (100 units/ml) in the line and leave capped for 2 h. Repeat step #1

2. Heparin may promote a low level thrombolytic state, thereby freeing the catheter. If infusion of essential medication is required, a new peripheral line should be started.

3. Obtain "catheterogram" x-ray in radiology suite

3. Injection of contrast through the catheter can demonstrate fibrin sheath radiographically and confirm catheter position.

4. Have epinephrine 0.3 ml 1:1000 dilution and IV hydrocortisone and diphenhydramine available at bedside. Mix streptokinase 250,000 units in 2 ml NS. Instill 2.5 ml in single-lumen Hickman catheter or, for double catheter, 1.5 ml in Hickman line and 1.0 ml in Broviac line. Clamp for 2 h. Aspirate until free return of blood is obtained and discard (do not flush). Continue routine care

4. Close attention to possible anaphylaxis is necessary since this occurs in 2.5% of patients exposed to streptokinase. Prompt treatment with epinephrine, hydrocortisone, and/or diphenhydramine (Benadryl) can prevent serious sequelae (see Streptokinase Infusion, pp. 188–189).

INTUBATION OF THE TRACHEA

Intubation of the trachea will protect the airways from major aspiration as well as permit mechanical ventilation and administration of controlled amounts of oxygen. The procedure may be performed orally or nasally, although the latter is contraindicated in facial or head trauma. Complications include sinusitis, laryngeal damage, and intubation of the esophagus. Endotracheal tube size is important only in rare circumstances.

PRE-INTUBATION

1. Diet: NPO	1. Routine.
2. Suction at bedside	2. Routine.
3. Intubation tray with resuscitation cart available	3. Resuscitation equipment should always be present and should include muscle relaxants as well as antiarrhythmic medications.

POST-INTUBATION

1. Secure tube at 22 cm at the teeth	1. This is generally the correct length of insertion.
2. Check ET tube for CO_2	2. An immediate check for expired CO_2 levels with a portable CO_2 meter assures tracheal intubation.
3. Portable CXR for tube placement	3. A chest x-ray for confirmation of endotracheal tube position is needed to check for the possibility of mainstem bronchus intubation.
4. Routine care, including cuff pressure checks, q shift	4. By maintaining low cuff pressures, many complications (including tracheal erosion) can be avoided or minimized.

LIVER BIOPSY

Percutaneous liver biopsy is performed to sample liver tissue to determine the histologic type of hepatitis, diagnose granulomatous liver disease, and look for malignancy. Liver biopsy can also be done under direct vision by peritoneoscopy, during which multiple biopsies can be performed.

PRE-LIVER BIOPSY ORDERS

1. Diet: NPO after midnight	1. Routine.
2. Premedications: None	2. Premedication is usually not required. Occasionally, a patient may request or need prebiopsy sedation. However, with percutaneous biopsy, it is essential that the patient be alert and cooperative.

3. Laboratory: PT, platelet count, bleeding time, Hct

3. These studies are routine for most biopsy procedures. If there is a high suspicion of a clotting abnormality, a coagulation screening test, including PTT, PT, and fibrinogen, in addition to other studies, may be indicated.

POST-LIVER BIOPSY ORDERS

1. Vital Signs: Pulse and BP q 1 h × 6, then q 2 h for next 18 h when awake
   Call physician if there is a > 20 mm Hg drop in systolic BP

1. Vital signs are monitored primarily for evidence of bleeding. The patient's hematocrit level may be checked the following morning.

2. Activity: Bed rest for 24 h

2. The patient's activity should be minimal to prevent bleeding.

LUMBAR PUNCTURE (LP)

The lumbar puncture is performed to sample the cerebrospinal fluid (CSF) for evidence of infection, bleeding, malignancy, or raised intracranial pressure. Lumbar puncture is a common ward and outpatient test and usually requires no pre-procedure orders. The necessary equipment should be readily available, however. In addition, patients with suspected raised intracranial pressure who might be susceptible to transtentorial herniation of intracranial contents when the subarachnoid space is entered should be examined for that possibility by other means (usually by a CT scan if available) prior to LP, or LP must be performed with extreme caution using the smallest possible spinal needle.

POST-LUMBAR PUNCTURE ORDERS

1. Activity: Patient to lie prone for 1 h; absolute bed rest for 12 h after the procedure

2. Nursing: Call physician if patient develops a headache

1–2. The most common complication of lumbar puncture is a post-LP headache, which has been reported in over 20% of patients. The headache is caused by a leak of CSF at the site of the lumbar puncture. Careful technique, the use of narrow-gauge needles, and bed rest in a prone position after LP minimize the likelihood of this complication.

MECHANICAL VENTILATION

Mechanical ventilation allows control of both oxygenation and carbon dioxide excretion. Many sophisticated ventilators are available, but most of the essential features are not complicated. The mode of ventilation (e.g., control, assisted mandatory ventilation [AMV], intermittent mandatory ventilation [IMV]) has received much attention but is usually less important than other settings. The key settings are tidal volume, rate per minute, and inspired oxygen concentration (FiO_2). Complications of mechanical ventilation include the "auto-PEEP" phenomenon in patients with airflow obstruction; cardiovascular compromise, especially in volume depleted patients; and barotrauma if excessive tidal volumes are used.

1. Endotracheal tube placed	1. Routine.

2. Begin mechanical ventilation
   a. Mode: AMV
	2. Routine
	   a. AMV is the preferred mode in respiratory failure, although some clinicians prefer IMV especially for weaning.

b. Tidal Volume: 750 ml (10 ml/kg)	b. A tidal volume over 7.5 ml/kg will avoid microatelectasis; a tidal volume less than 12 ml/kg will cause less barotrauma.
c. Rate: 12/min	c. The rate is adjusted to keep the average minute ventilation adequate for near normal pH and may be adjusted on the basis of pCO_2 measured in arterial blood gases.
d. FiO_2: Initially 100%. Use ear oximeter and taper FiO_2 until % Sat = 93%–95%, then check ABG's for confirmation	d. Oxygen toxicity can be avoided by keeping the FiO_2 below 60%. Use of an oximeter minimizes the need for ABGs. Other settings (peak flow, inspiration/expiration ratios, and so forth) will depend largely on various clinical conditions.

PACEMAKER INSERTION

Short-term pacing of the heart is often indicated in conditions with varying degrees of urgency. The transvenous approach (femoral, subclavian, internal jugular, antecubital) is employed most commonly, especially in situations that have not yet reached a critical stage. The transthoracic or transcutaneous approach is used in absolute emergencies requiring immediate pacing. However, a second transvenous pacer should be placed as soon as possible after transthoracic placement or transcutaneous pacing.

Short-term pacing using the transvenous route can be maintained for up to 6 weeks. Patients should be in an intensive care unit, and the indication for the pacemaker should be clearly specified to the nursing staff. The following orders are used following successful insertion of a transvenous pacemaker:

1. Nursing:
   a. Local care: Change dressing and apply antibacterial ointment to entry site every day

   b. Continuous ECG; watch for failure of pacemaker to capture, sense, or fire; check threshold q shift

   c. Record pacemaker setting:
      Rate: 70
      Mode: Demand
      MEV: 5 mA
      Threshold: 0.5 mA

   a. Routine wound care should be performed to prevent infection.

   b. Pacemaker failure should be detected early and may be suspected if the heart slows or capture does not occur for the indicated rate.

   c. The rate, mode (demand or fixed), and output of the pacemaker should be ordered so that the actual settings are checked and recorded. Pacing threshold at the time of insertion should generally be ≤ 1 mA.

PARACENTESIS

Paracentesis of ascites fluid is usually performed for diagnostic purposes. In general, no pre- or post-procedure orders are required.

PERCUTANEOUS TRANSLUMINAL CORONARY ANGIOPLASTY (PTCA)

Percutaneous transluminal coronary angioplasty, or PTCA, has been used increasingly for patients with segmental obstructive coronary artery disease as an alternative to coronary artery bypass surgery. The indications vary considerably in different regions and with different operators. The cardiac surgeons should be aware of all patients undergoing PTCA, and the patient and hospital staff should be prepared for immediate coronary artery surgery in the event of a complication or failure of PTCA.

PRE-ANGIOPLASTY ORDERS

1. Nursing: Prepare the groin or arm; have the patient take pHisoHex showers × 3, and have the patient void before procedure; IV heparin lock, lt. arm

2. Diet: NPO except medications with small sips of water after midnight

3. Medications:
   PM before PTCA:
   Aspirin 325 mg PO hs

1. Routine; pHisoHex showers are taken in preparation for anticipated coronary bypass surgery.

2. If the procedure is scheduled in the afternoon, the patient can have a clear liquid breakfast.

3. Antiplatelet therapy is generally begun the night before PTCA. If the right coronary

Triazolam 0.25 mg PO hs prn for sleep; may repeat × 1

On call: (After consent obtained)

Lorazepam 2 mg PO

Meperidine 75 mg, promethazine 15 mg IM

artery is to be dilated, some physicians would also give atropine 0.8 mg IM on call. Cardiologists often prefer starting therapy with a calcium channel blocker (usually nifedipine or diltiazem) before PTCA to reduce the risk of coronary arterial spasm.

4. Laboratory:
Type and hold 6 units whole blood, three 10 ml red top tubes for possible coronary bypass surgery

4. Routine.

POST-ANGIOPLASTY ORDERS

1. Vital Signs: Check BP, heart rate, and distal pulses q 30 min × 2, q 1 h × 2, then q 4 h × 24 h if condition is stable

Call physician if:

Systolic BP < 100 or > 160

Pulse > 120 or < 60

Decrease in peripheral pulses, hematoma, or extremity or chest pain occurs

1. Changes in vital signs may indicate a complication of the procedure, such as blood loss or occlusion of a dilated artery.

2. Activity:
Bed rest for 8 hours after arterial line is pulled. May elevate head of bed ≤ 30 degrees

2. In complicated cases or where an intimal tear or dissection is suspected, the arterial sheath may be left in place for 12–24 hours until the patient's condition is clearly stable. Restriction of activity can help prevent local bleeding at the puncture site.

3. Nursing: Flush heparin lock q shift with 10 units heparin irrigation solution

3. Routine.

4. Diet: Resume previous diet order

4. Routine.

5. Medications:
Codeine 30–60 mg PO q 3–4 h prn arteriotomy or cutdown site pain

Aspirin 325 mg PO on return, then qd

Nifedipine 10 mg PO q 6 h

Resume other previous medications

5. Antiplatelet and calcium channel blockade are used to preserve patency of the dilated vessel. Patients on an alternate calcium channel blocking drug could have this drug restarted instead of using nifedipine.

6. Special:
Foley catheter I and O if unable to void in 6 h or prn

6. May help improve patient comfort.

RENAL BIOPSY

Percutaneous renal biopsy is performed to determine pathology of kidney disease. It is most useful in classifying the glomerulonephritides. The tissue is usually examined by light and electron microscopy and with immunofluorescent staining.

PRE-RENAL BIOPSY ORDERS

1. Diet: Clear liquids for meal immediately preceding biopsy

1. Routine.

2. Laboratory: Hct, PT, platelet count; type and crossmatch for 2 units whole blood

2. Bleeding is the most serious complication of renal biopsy and is frequent and severe enough to justify routinely having blood ready in the blood bank.

POST-RENAL BIOPSY ORDERS

1. Vital Signs: BP, Pulse, Resp q 15 min × 2 h, q 30 min × 2 h, q 1 h × 4 h, then q 2 h × 16 h; Temp q 2 h × 8 h, then q 4 h × 16 h
Call physician if:
BP < 90 systolic
Temp > 38°C

1–5. All postbiopsy orders are designed to detect and minimize bleeding from the biopsy site.

2. Activity: Strict bed rest lying flat for 24 h

3. Diet: Clear liquids 4 h after biopsy

4. Medications: No ASA or NSAID

5. Laboratory: Hct 4 and 8 h after biopsy and in AM; collect urine sequentially in containers labeled with the time of collection; spin Hct on urine if bloody
Call physician if:
Hct drops 3%
Patient has hematuria

SWAN-GANZ CATHETER (FLOW-DIRECTED PULMONARY ARTERY CATHETER)

Swan-Ganz catheters are used to monitor pulmonary artery (PA) and pulmonary wedge pressure in shock from any cause and during administration of intravenous afterload therapy. They may also be used when heart failure is suspected but not a certainty. The route of entry is influenced by the urgency of the situation. The antecubital, subclavian, internal jugular, or femoral veins may be used. Fluoroscopy should be employed if it is available and the patient's condition permits. Patients should be in an intensive care unit.

The following orders are indicated following placement of a Swan-Ganz catheter:

1. Nursing:
   a. Local care: Change dressing and apply antibiotic ointment to site every day
   b. Heparin flush (2 ml of heparin per 500 ml D5W): Place on continuous infusion system of 3 ml/h
   c. Continuous monitoring of PA port
   d. Call physician if PA becomes permanently "wedged," if catheter slips back into right ventricle, or if wedge readings cease
   e. Record PA, wedge, and RA pressures q 2 h or as needed clinically; cardiac output determinations q shift or as indicated if available

1. Routine wound care should be performed to prevent infection. Many ICUs have standard procedures for monitoring Swan-Ganz catheters.

2. Laboratory: CXR

2. Chest x-ray is routine to check line placement and to rule out pneumothorax.

THORACENTESIS

Thoracentesis is performed for diagnostic purposes (to sample pleural fluid) or for therapeutic purposes (to remove pleural fluid causing respiratory difficulty). Usually, no pre-procedure orders are required, although decubitus chest films should be taken to be certain that the fluid is free-flowing. If the patient has a suspected bleeding tendency, or if a pleural biopsy is planned, the PT, platelet count, and hematocrit should be checked.

POST-THORACENTESIS ORDERS

1. Laboratory: CXR—PA, inspiration and expiration—indication: pneumothorax

1. A chest x-ray is routine after thoracentesis to rule out a pneumothorax. Unless complications have occurred, the nursing care and monitoring of vital signs need not be altered.

THROMBOLYTIC THERAPY FOR ACUTE MYOCARDIAL INFARCTION: STREPTOKINASE INFUSION, TISSUE PLASMINOGEN ACTIVATOR (TPA) INFUSION

Intravenous infusion of thrombolytic agents shortly after the onset of chest pain in patients having an acute myocardial infarction can result in restoration of coronary artery blood flow in 50–70% of cases. Patients should be considered for this therapy if they are less than 75 years old, and have ECG evidence of an acute infarction believed to be less than 6 hours old. Contraindications include conditions precluding use of anticoagulation (active peptic ulcer disease, disseminated malignancy, retinopathy, hypertension with diastolic BP > 120 mm Hg), a recent major surgical procedure (< 2 weeks) or neurosurgical procedure or stroke (< 4 weeks), recent CPR, and recent subclavian vein or arterial puncture (except with small-gauge needles for ABG determination).

STREPTOKINASE INFUSION

Although controversy exists as to which thrombolytic agent is superior in the treatment of acute myocardial infarction, streptokinase is preferred at most centers because of its significantly reduced cost. It should not be administered to patients with a history of prior exposure to streptokinase.

1. Admission orders for myocardial infarction apply

   1. Routine.

2. Establish at least 2 16–18-gauge IV lines with D5W at TKO

   2. Future laboratory tests need to be obtained without venipuncture.

3. Draw baseline CBC, coagulation screen, CPK with MB isoenzyme, electrolytes, and an additional tube to type and hold 2 units of packed red blood cells.

   3. Following streptokinase infusion, the intense fibrinolytic state will prevent adequate measurement of the blood coagulation profile.

4. Premedication:
   ASA 325 mg PO chewed
   Diphenhydramine 50 mg IV push
   Hydrocortisone 100 mg IV push
   Nitroglycerin 0.3 mg sublingually

   4. Anaphylaxis occurs in 2.5% of patients and can be prevented or attenuated by use of premedication. Consider intravenous nitroglycerin and/or morphine for persistent pain and intravenous beta-blocker therapy.

5. Infuse 1.5 million units of streptokinase in 100–250 ml D5W or saline over 1 h. Observe patient closely for any signs of anaphylaxis

   5. Signs of anaphylaxis include Bp change of > 25 mm Hg, rash, musculoskeletal pain, flushing, itching, fever or chill, nausea, bronchospasm, and periorbital edema or an-

gioedema. The administration of heparin after streptokinase infusion is controversial. If used, heparin, 1000 units/h, should be started 2 h after streptokinase infusion and adjusted to maintain the PTT 1.5–2.0 × control.

6. Laboratory:
   CPK with MB every 6 h × 24 h
   Tomorrow: CBC, UA, guaiac stools, ECG, CXR

TISSUE PLASMINOGEN ACTIVATOR (TPA) INFUSION

1. Admission orders for myocardial infarction apply

1. Routine.

2. Establish at least 2 16–18-gauge IV lines with D5W at TKO

2. Future laboratory tests need to be obtained without venipuncture. Some clinicians prefer establishing an arterial line prior to initiation of thrombolytic therapy. However, placement of an arterial line should not unduly delay the start of thrombolytic therapy.

3. Draw baseline CBC, platelets, electrolytes, coagulation screen, CPK with MB isoenzyme, and an additional tube to type and hold 2 units of packed red blood cells

3. Following TPA infusion, the intense fibrinolytic state will prevent adequate measurement of the blood coagulation profile.

4. Premedication:
   ASA 325 mg PO chewed
   Nitroglycerin 0.3 mg sublingually

5. Infuse TPA 60 mg IV over first hour followed by 40 mg IV over the next hour

6. After 1 h of TPA infusion, begin heparin 5000 units IV bolus followed by 500–1000 units/h IV

6. Heparin should be administered at a rate to maintain PTT at 1.5–2.0 × control. (INR = 2.0–3.0)

7. Laboratory:
   CPK with MB every 6 h × 24 h
   PTT 2 h after TPA infusion
   Tomorrow: CBC, UA, guaiac stools, ECG, CXR

7. Close attention for possible sites of bleeding should be maintained for 48–72 h.

PART IV

THERAPEUTIC AGENTS

Specific information on over 500 drugs is included in this section, which is intended to be a convenient, practical, and up-to-date source for the busy student, resident, and practicing physician. We have selected drugs used for hospitalized as well as ambulatory patients. Admittedly, our selection of drugs is somewhat eclectic, since a comprehensive listing of all available drugs with indications, side effects, and drug interactions is not feasible. Nevertheless, we have tried to include commonly used drugs and the most essential prescribing information.

The organization of this section follows the topic headings of Part II, namely, a listing of drugs by major organs and systems (e.g., Cardiovascular Drugs, Dermatologic Drugs, Endocrine Drugs). The part entitled "Care and Comfort Drugs" includes preparations that do not fall under specific organ disease categories (e.g., analgesics, cough preparations, hypnotics, laxatives, and sedatives).

Drugs are listed in a tabular format. The first column lists the generic name. "Trade Name" is the heading of the second column. Under this heading, the availability of generic forms is indicated, and multiple trade names are often specified by "and others" following selected common trade names. The third column notes the routes of administration (IV, IM, PO, and SC) and the dosage of oral preparations. Many of the drugs are available in liquid preparations for patients unable to swallow pills. The concentrations of IM and IV preparations are not listed since the physician seldom requires this information for prescribing. The fourth column describes the general indications for use of the drugs. The usual dosages are listed in the fifth column, and the sixth column, labeled "Cautions/Comments," includes major side effects, contraindications, and other pertinent information.

In general, fixed-combination drugs are not listed, as we believe that the use of these types of drugs should be discouraged. Exceptions are some analgesic combinations that may have synergistic effects and commonly used combinations (e.g., Lomotil).

The pharmacologic world is ever changing, and pharmacologic references should be consulted for the most recent indications, dosages, and side effects. This is especially important for drugs that are unfamiliar to the prescribing physician. We have drawn upon a large number of sources for the information in this section, including the *United States Pharmacopeia,* the *AMA Drug Evaluations,* the *Physicians' Desk Reference,* the *American Hospital Formulary Service Drug Information,* and the *Blue Book of Pharmacologic Therapeutics* (Gordon Johnson).

ALL DOSAGES LISTED ARE FOR ADULTS ONLY.

CARE AND COMFORT DRUGS

GENERIC NAME	TRADE NAME	PREPARATIONS	GENERAL INDICATIONS	USUAL DOSAGE	CAUTIONS/COMMENTS
Analgesics					
Acetaminophen	Tylenol Datril Others	PO: 60, 300, 325, 500, 600 mg tab 325, 500 mg cap Suppository: 125, 500, 600, 650, 900 mg	Mild pain Antipyretic	PO: 650 mg every 4 h	Large doses (15 g) may cause severe hepatic damage Rate of absorption of suppositories varies among different brands
Aspirin	Many brands	PO: 65, 75, 80, 325, 500, 650, 800 mg tab	Mild pain Antipyretic Antiinflammatory	PO: 650 mg every 4–6 h	May cause GI distress Suppositories are available but not recommended owing to variable absorption Antiinflammatory therapeutic blood level is 10–25 mg/dl. Analgesic level is lower
Codeine		IM PO: 15, 30, 60 mg tab	Mild to moderate pain Useful antitussive	IM, PO: 30–60 mg every 4–6 h	Addiction
Diclofenac	Voltaren	PO: 25, 50, 75 mg tab	Mild to moderate pain	PO: 50–75 mg every 8–12 h	GI side effects
Diflunisal	Dolobid	PO: 250, 500 mg tab	Mild to moderate pain	PO: 1 g followed by 500 mg every 12 h	GI side effects are less than with aspirin
Fenoprofen	Nalfon	PO: 200, 300 mg cap 600 mg tab	Mild to moderate pain	PO: 200 mg every 4–6 h	GI side effects

Table continued on following page

GENERIC NAME	TRADE NAME	PREPARATIONS	GENERAL INDICATIONS	USUAL DOSAGE	CAUTIONS/COMMENTS
Hydromorphone	Dilaudid Generic	IV IM SC PO: 1, 2, 3, 4 mg tab Suppository: 3 mg	Severe pain	IV: 1-5 mg IV slowly every 4–6 h IM, SC: 1–1.5 mg (up to 4 mg) every 4–6 h PO: 2 mg every 4–6 h	Respiratory depression Addiction
Ibuprofen	Advil Motrin Rufen	PO: 300, 400, 600 mg tab	Mild to moderate pain	PO: 400 mg every 4–6 h	200 mg size available OTC (Advil)
Ketoprofen	Orudis	PO: 25, 50, 75 mg cap	Moderate to severe pain	PO: 50–75 mg every 6–8 h	GI side effects
Ketorolac	Toradol	IM	Moderate to severe pain	IM: 30–60 mg as loading dose, then 15–30 mg every 6 h	Possible GI side effects
Levorphanol	Levo-Dromoran	PO: 2 mg tab SQ	Severe pain	PO/SQ: 2 mg every 6–8 h	Addiction Sedation Respiratory depression
Meclofenamate	Meclomen	PO: 50, 100 mg cap	Mild to moderate pain	PO: 50–100 mg every 8 h	GI side effects
Meperidine	Demerol Generic	IV IM SC PO: 50, 100 mg tab	Severe pain	IV: 50–150 mg slowly every 3–4 h IM, SC: 50–150 mg every 3–4 h PO: 50–150 mg every 3–4 h	Respiratory depression Addiction
Methadone	Dolophine	IM PO: 5, 10, 40 mg tab	Narcotic detoxification programs Severe pain	IM: 2.5–10 mg PO: 2.5–10 mg every 6–8 h or daily for detoxification programs	Dosage must be individualized. Often used as part of a "pain cocktail"

Generic	Brand	Dosage Forms	Uses	Dosage	Nursing Considerations
Morphine		IV IM SC PO: 10, 15, 30 mg tab	Severe pain (myocardial infarction, renal colic) Pulmonary edema	IV: 2–10 mg slowly over several min every 4–6 h IM, SC: 5–20 mg every 4–6 h	Respiratory depression Addiction Oral route is one-sixth as potent as other routes; not routinely used but may be of benefit for cancer pain
Nalbuphine	Nubain	IV IM SC	Severe pain	IV: 2–10 mg slowly over several min every 3–6 h IM, SC: 10 mg every 3–6 h	Respiratory depression Addiction Equivalent to morphine on a milligram basis
Naproxen	Naprosyn	PO: 250, 375, 500 mg tab	Mild to moderate pain	PO: 500 mg initially, then 250 mg 3 times daily	GI side effects
Oxymorphone	Numorphan	IV IM SC Suppository: 5 mg	Severe pain	IV: 0.5 mg initially IM, SC: 0.5–1.5 mg every 4–6 h	Respiratory depression Addiction
Pentazocine	Talwin Talwin NX (oral)	IV IM SC PO: 50 mg tab	Moderate to severe pain	IV, IM, SC: 30 mg every 3–4 h PO: 50–100 mg every 3–4 h	Addiction Avoid subcutaneous route if possible because of possible tissue damage
Phenazopyridine	Pyridium	PO: 100, 200 mg tab	Urinary tract infections (pain, burning, urgency symptoms)	PO: 200 mg 3 times daily	Should be discontinued when symptoms subside Urine is discolored orange
Piroxicam	Feldene	PO: 10, 20 mg cap	Mild to moderate pain	PO: 20 mg every 24 h	GI side effects
Propoxyphene HCl	Darvon Dolene SK-65 Generic	PO: 32, 65 mg cap	Mild pain	PO: 65 mg 3–4 times daily	Potentially addicting Caution patient about use with other CNS depressants, including alcohol

Table continued on following page

GENERIC NAME	TRADE NAME	PREPARATIONS	GENERAL INDICATIONS	USUAL DOSAGE	CAUTIONS/COMMENTS
Propoxyphene napsylate	Darvon-N	PO: 100 mg tab	Mild pain	PO: 100 mg 3–4 times daily	Potentially addicting Caution patient about use with other CNS depressants, including alcohol
Sulindac	Clinoril	PO: 150, 200 mg tab	Mild to moderate pain	PO: 150–200 mg every 12 h	GI side effects
Suprofen	Suprol	PO: 200 mg cap	Mild to moderate pain	PO: 200 mg every 4–6 h	Because of renal toxicity, should be considered a second line drug
Tolmetin	Tolectin	PO: 400 mg cap; 200, 600 mg tab	Mild to moderate pain	PO: 400 mg every 8 h	GI side effects

ANALGESIC DOSAGE EQUIVALENT TO 10 MG MORPHINE

	IM, IV	PO
Morphine	10 mg	60 mg
Codeine	130 mg	200 mg
Hydromorphone (Dilaudid)	1.5 mg	7.5 mg
Meperidine (Demerol)	100 mg	400 mg
Nalbuphine (Nubain)	10 mg	N.A.
Oxymorphone (Numorphan)	1.5 mg	N.A.
Pentazocine (Talwin)	60 mg	180 mg

GENERIC NAME	TRADE NAME	PREPARATIONS	GENERAL INDICATIONS	USUAL DOSAGE	CAUTIONS/COMMENTS
Analgesic Combinations					
Codeine, aspirin	Empirin with codeine #1, 2, 3, 4 Ascodeen-30 (equivalent to Empirin with codeine #3)	PO: Tab, contains 325 mg aspirin and 7.5 mg codeine (#1) or 15 mg codeine (#2) or 30 mg codeine (#3) or 60 mg codeine (#4)	Moderate pain	PO: 1 tab every 4–6 h	See *Aspirin*, *Codeine*
Codeine, acetaminophen	Tylenol with codeine Phenaphen with codeine Empracet with codeine	PO: Tab, contains 300 mg acetaminophen and 7.5 mg codeine (#1) or 15 mg codeine (#2) or 30 mg codeine (#3) or 60 mg codeine (#4)	Moderate pain	PO: 1 tab every 4–6 h	Phenaphen with codeine contains 325 mg acetaminophen
Oxycodone, acetaminophen	Percocet	PO: Tab contains 5 mg oxycodone and 325 mg acetaminophen	Moderate to severe pain	PO: 1 tab every 6 h	Potentially addicting
Oxycodone, aspirin	Percodan Percodan-Demi	PO: Tab, contains 4.5 mg oxycodone and 325 mg aspirin	Moderate to severe pain	PO: 1 tab every 6 h	Potentially addicting Percodan-demi contains ½ the amount of oxycodone
Propoxyphene, acetaminophen	Wygesic	PO: Tab, contains 65 mg propoxyphene and 650 mg acetaminophen	Mild to moderate pain	PO: 1 tab every 6 h	See *Propoxyphene HCl* under *Analgesics*
Propoxyphene, aspirin	Darvon with ASA	PO: Tab, contains 65 mg propoxyphene and 325 mg aspirin	Mild to moderate pain	PO: 1 tab every 4–6 h	See *Propoxyphene HCl* under *Analgesics*

Table continued on following page

GENERIC NAME	TRADE NAME	PREPARATIONS	GENERAL INDICATIONS	USUAL DOSAGE	CAUTIONS/COMMENTS
Propoxyphene napsylate, acetaminophen	Darvocet-N	PO: Tab, contains 100 mg propoxyphene napsylate and 650 mg acetaminophen	Mild to moderate pain	PO: 1 tab every 6 h	See *Propoxyphene napsylate* under *Analgesics*
Propoxyphene napsylate, aspirin	Darvon-N with ASA	PO: Tab, contains 100 mg propoxyphene napsylate and 325 mg aspirin	Mild to moderate pain	PO: 1 tab every 4–6 h	See *Propoxyphene napsylate* under *Analgesics*
Antihistamines					
Astemizole	Hismanal	PO: 10 mg tab	Allergic rhinitis	PO: 10 mg every 24 h	Less sedating May prolong QT interval
Brompheniramine	Dimetane Generic	IV IM SM PO: 4 mg tab 8, 12 mg timed-release tab	Allergic rhinitis	IV, IM, SC: 5–20 mg PO: 4–8 mg 3–4 times daily 8 or 12 mg timed-release twice daily	Drowsiness
Chlorpheniramine	Chlor-Trimeton Histaspan Teldrin Generic	IV IM SC PO: 4 mg tab 8, 12 mg timed-release tab and cap	Allergic rhinitis Pruritus	IV, IM, SC: 5–20 mg PO: 4–8 mg 3–4 times daily 8 or 12 mg timed-release twice daily	Drowsiness 4 and 8 mg tablets are nonprescription
Cyproheptadine	Periactin	PO: 4 mg tab	Pruritus Cold urticaria	PO: 4–20 mg daily in divided doses	Drowsiness Weight gain Dosage must be individualized

Drug	Brand/Generic	Preparations	Indications	Dosage	Comments
Diphenhydramine	Benadryl Generic	IV IM PO: 25, 50 mg cap	Allergic reactions Dystonic reactions to phenothiazines	IV, IM: 50 mg (maximum 400 mg daily) PO: 25–50 mg 3–4 times daily	Drowsiness IM injections should be deep 25 mg tablets are nonprescription
Pyrilamine maleate	Generic	PO: 25, 50 mg tab	Allergic rhinitis	PO: 25–50 mg 3–4 times daily	Drowsiness
Terfenadine	Seldane	PO: 60 mg tab	Allergic rhinitis	PO: 60 mg twice daily	Less sedating May prolong QT interval
Tripelennamine	Pyribenzamine Generic	PO: 25, 50 mg tab	Allergic rhinitis	PO: 50 mg 3–4 times daily	Drowsiness
Triprolidine	Actidil	PO: 2.5 mg tab	Allergic rhinitis	PO: 2.5 mg 2–3 times daily	Drowsiness
Numerous other antihistamines are available					
Antihistamine Combinations					
Brompheniramine, phenylephrine, phenylpropanolamine	Dimetapp	PO: Tab, timed-release, contains 12 mg, 15 mg, and 15 mg, respectively, of generic ingredients	URI, sinus symptoms	PO: 1 tab twice daily	Drowsiness
Chlorpheniramine, phenylpropanolamine, isopropamide	Ornade	PO: Cap, timed-release, contains 8 mg, 50 mg, and 2.5 mg, respectively, of generic ingredients	URI, sinus symptoms	PO: 1 cap twice daily	Drowsiness
Triprolidine, pseudoephedrine	Actifed	PO: Tab contains 2.5 mg triprolidine and 60 mg pseudoephedrine	URI, sinus symptoms	PO: 1 tab 3–4 times daily	Drowsiness Available OTC
Numerous other antihistamine-containing mixtures are available					

Table continued on following page

GENERIC NAME	TRADE NAME	PREPARATIONS	GENERAL INDICATIONS	USUAL DOSAGE	CAUTIONS/COMMENTS
Cough Preparations					
Codeine	Generic	PO: 15, 30, 60 mg tab	Moderate to severe cough	PO: 15–30 mg every 4–6 h as necessary	Addiction with prolonged use
Dextromethorphan	Generic	PO: Syrup, 7.5 and 15 mg/5 ml	Mild cough	PO: 15–30 mg 3–4 times daily	Nonnarotic cough suppressant
Guaifenesin	Robitussin Generic	PO: Liquid, 100 mg/5 ml	Mild cough	PO: 1 tsp (5 ml) every 3–4 h	Expectorant
Numerous other cough drugs and combinations are available					
Decongestants					
Pseudoephedrine	Novafed Sudafed Others	PO: 30, 60 mg tab	Nasal congestion	PO: 60 mg 3 or 4 times daily	30 mg size available OTC
Numerous other decongestants are available					
Hypnotics					
Chloral hydrate	Generic	PO: 225, 250, 450, 500 mg cap Suppository	Hypnotic Sedative	As hypnotic: 1 g at bedtime As sedative: 250–500 mg 3 times daily	Reduce dosage in severe renal or hepatic disease
Flurazepam	Dalmane	PO: 15, 30 mg cap	Hypnotic	PO: 15–30 mg at bedtime	Ataxia, vertigo Paradoxical excitation may occur
Pentobarbital	Nembutal Generic	IV IM PO: 30, 50, 100 mg cap 90, 100 mg timed-release tab	Hypnotic Sedative	As hypnotic, until effect is achieved (maximum 500 mg) IV: 100 mg initially, then small increments IM: 150–250 mg	Avoid in elderly patients, if possible Effectiveness may be lost with continued use

Generic	Brand	Formulation	Use	Dosage	Comments
Secobarbital	Seconal	IV IM PO: 30, 50, 100 mg cap Suppository: 30, 60, 120, 200 mg	Hypnotic	IV: 100 mg (slowly) IM: 100 mg PO: 100 mg at bedtime As sedative: PO: 30 mg 3–4 times daily or 1 timed-release tab daily	Avoid in elderly patients, if possible Effectiveness may be lost with continued use
Temazepam	Restoril	PO: 15, 30 mg cap	Hypnotic	PO: 15–30 mg at bedtime	
Triazolam	Halcion	PO: 0.125, 0.25, 0.5 mg	Hypnotic	PO: 0.25–0.5 mg at bedtime	Half dose in elderly
Laxatives Bisacodyl	Dulcolax Generic	PO: 5 mg tab Suppository: 10 mg	Constipation	PO: 5 mg twice daily Suppository: 1 daily	Tablet should not be taken with milk or antacids
Cascara	Generic	PO: 300 mg tab, fluid extract, liquid, powder	Constipation	PO: 200–400 mg of extract daily or 1 tab daily	Brown to reddish discoloration of urine
Docusate sodium	Colace Dialose Generic	PO: 50, 100 mg cap (Colace) 100, 250 mg cap (generic)	Constipation	PO: 50–250 mg daily (usual: 100 mg cap daily)	Wetting agents; may take 48 h for effect Nonprescription
Glycerine suppositories		Suppository: 3 g	Constipation	Suppository: 1 g as needed	
Lactulose	Chronulac	PO: Syrup	Constipation	PO: 30 ml (2 tbsp) daily	Effect is often delayed 48 h Use with caution in diabetic patients, as it contains lactose and galactose
Magnesium citrate		PO: Liquid	Constipation	PO: 100–200 ml	Nonprescription
Milk of magnesia		PO: Liquid	Constipation	PO: 15–30 ml daily	Nonprescription

Table continued on following page

GENERIC NAME	TRADE NAME	PREPARATIONS	GENERAL INDICATIONS	USUAL DOSAGE	CAUTIONS/COMMENTS
Psyllium hydrophilic colloid	Effersyllium Konsyl Metamucil Others	PO: Powder	Constipation	PO: 1 tsp or 1 packet in glass of water or juice 1–3 times daily	Bulk-forming agent; may take several days for effect to be achieved Nonprescription
Sodium phosphate	Fleet enema	Enema: 4 oz	Constipation	Enema: 4 oz as needed	Nonprescription
Numerous other laxatives and combinations are available					
Sedatives: See *Antianxiety Agents* for Benzodiazepines (pp. 269–270)					
Amobarbital	Amytal Generic	IV IM PO: 15, 30, 50, 100 mg tab 65, 200 mg cap	Sedative Hypnotic Severe agitation	As sedative: PO: 30–60 mg 2–3 times daily As hypnotic: IM, IV: 130–200 mg at bedtime For severe agitation: IM, IV: 130–260 mg (up to 500 mg)	Respiratory depression at high doses
Chloral hydrate	See under *Hypnotics*				
Phenobarbital	Luminal Solfoton Generic	IV IM PO: 7.5, 15, 30, 60, 100 mg Suppository: 60 mg	Sedative Anticonvulsant Hypnotic	As sedative: IM, IV: 30–60 mg 2–3 times daily PO: 30 mg 2–3 times daily As hypnotic: IM, IV: 100–320 mg PO: 100–320 mg	Oral route is preferred for sedative In high dosages, may be used as hypnotic and anticonvulsant
Pentobarbital	See under *Hypnotics*				

ANTINEOPLASTIC DRUGS

Antineoplastic drugs should be prescribed only by physicians who are familiar with their use. The art of treating neoplasms is changing so rapidly that consultation with experienced physicians is recommended. Virtually all antineoplastic agents cause acute toxicity (nausea and vomiting) and delayed toxicity (bone marrow depression). Dosages listed are representative of those found in various chemotherapy regimens and may vary considerably in practice.

GENERIC NAME	TRADE NAME	PREPARATIONS	GENERAL INDICATIONS	USUAL DOSAGE	CAUTIONS / COMMENTS
Alkylating Agents					
Busulfan	Myleran	PO: 2 mg tab	Chronic myelogenous leukemia Polycythemia vera	PO: 4–8 mg daily until leukocyte count falls 50% or to 10,000 Usual maintenance dose: 2–4 mg	Bone marrow depression Pulmonary fibrosis Amenorrhea Hyperpigmentation of skin
Carmustine (BCNU)	BCNU	IV	CNS tumors Multiple myeloma Lymphomas	IV: 200 mg/M² every 4–6 weeks	Bone marrow depression Pulmonary fibrosis
Chlorambucil	Leukeran	PO: 2 mg tab	Chronic lymphocytic leukemia Hodgkin's disease Non-Hodgkin's lymphoma and other cancers	PO: 0.1–0.2 mg/kg daily for 3–6 weeks Usual maintenance dose: 0.03–0.1 mg/kg daily	Bone marrow depression Amenorrhea Pulmonary fibrosis
Cyclophosphamide	Cytoxan	IV PO: 25, 50 mg tab	Hodgkin's disease Non-Hodgkin's lymphoma and other cancers	PO, IV: 2–7.5 mg/kg daily for 10 days Adjust dose according to response Maintenance low-dose therapy may then be administered Other regimens are used	Bone marrow depression Alopecia (30% of patients) Hemorrhagic cystitis

Table continued on following page

GENERIC NAME	TRADE NAME	PREPARATIONS	GENERAL INDICATIONS	USUAL DOSAGE	CAUTIONS/COMMENTS
Dacarbazine	DTIC-Dome	IV	Melanoma Hodgkin's disease and other tumors	IV: 2–4.5 mg/kg daily for 10 days every 28 days	Bone marrow depression
Lomustine (CCNU)	CeeNU	PO: 10, 40, 100 mg cap	CNS tumors Hodgkin's disease and other tumors	PO: 130 mg/M² single dose every 6 weeks	Bone marrow depression
Mechlorethamine	Mustargen	IV	Hodgkin's disease and other lymphomas	IV: 6 mg/M² on days 1 and 8 as part of MOPP regimen; repeat every 28 days	Bone marrow depression Avoid extravasation
Melphalan	Alkeran	PO: 2 mg tab	Multiple myeloma Breast carcinoma Other tumors	PO: 0.25 mg/kg daily for 7 days, then maintenance therapy after 3 weeks Usual maintenance dose: 0.5–0.1 mg/kg daily Alternate regimen: 0.25 mg/kg daily for 4 days every 6 weeks	Bone marrow depression Amenorrhea
Thiotepa	Thiotepa	IV	Breast and ovarian carcinoma	IV: 0.2 mg/kg daily for 5 days every 4 weeks	Bone marrow depression
Antibiotics Bleomycin	Blenoxane	IV IM SC	Wilms' tumor Choriocarcinoma Testicular tumors and other tumors Squamous cell carcinomas Lymphomas	IV: 0.25–0.5 units/kg once or twice weekly	Pulmonary fibrosis Febrile reactions Stomatitis Skin eruptions

Drug	Brand	Route	Indication	Dosage	Toxicity
Dactinomycin (Actinomycin D)	Cosmegen	IV	Wilms' tumor Trophoblastic tumor Testicular tumor Ewing's sarcoma	IV: 0.5 mg daily for 5 days	Bone marrow depression Alopecia Avoid extravasation
Daunorubicin	Cerubidine	IV	Acute myelogenous leukemia	IV: 45 mg/M^2 daily for 3 days	Related to doxorubicin; usually used concurrently with other drugs Bone marrow depression Cardiomyopathy Stomatitis Alopecia Avoid extravasation
Doxorubicin	Adriamycin	IV	Acute lymphocytic and myelogenous leukemia and others	IV: 60–75 mg/M^2; repeat in 21 days	Alopecia Bone marrow depression Cardiomyopathy Avoid extravasation
Mitomycin	Mutamycin	IV	GI cancers and others	IV: 20 mg/M^2 in single dose every 6–8 weeks	Bone marrow depression Stomatitis Avoid extravasation
Plicamycin	Mithracin	IV	Testicular tumor	IV: 50 μg/kg every other day for 6 doses (slowly over 4–6 h)	Bleeding syndrome Bone marrow depression
Antimetabolites					
Cytarabine	Cytosar-U	IV IM	Acute myelogenous leukemia	IV: 2 mg/kg daily for 10 days IM: Maintenance dose: 1 mg/kg weekly	Bone marrow depression
Fluorouracil (5-FU)	Adrucil	IV	GI cancer Breast cancer	IV: 15 mg/kg weekly	Bone marrow depression

Table continued on following page

GENERIC NAME	TRADE NAME	PREPARATIONS	GENERAL INDICATIONS	USUAL DOSAGE	CAUTIONS/COMMENTS
Mercaptopurine	Purinethol	PO: 50 mg tab	Acute lymphocytic leukemia	PO: 2.5 mg/kg daily	Bone marrow depression
Methotrexate	Methotrexate Mexate	IV IM PO: 2.5 mg tab May also be given intrathecally	Trophoblastic tumors Testicular cancers Acute lymphocytic leukemia and other tumors	Numerous schedules are used	Bone marrow depression Alopecia Stomatitis Diarrhea
Thioguanine	Thioguanine	PO: 40 mg tab	Acute myelogenous leukemia	PO: 2 mg/kg daily	Bone marrow depression
Vinca Alkaloids					
Vinblastine	Velban	IV	Hodgkin's disease Lymphoma and other tumors Testicular cancer	IV: 4–8 mg/M^2 weekly Maintenance dose: 10 mg once or twice weekly	Bone marrow depression Alopecia Avoid extravasation
Vincristine	Oncovin	IV	Acute lymphocytic leukemia Lymphomas	IV: 1–2 mg/M^2 weekly	Bone marrow depression Alopecia Peripheral neuropathy Avoid extravasation
Miscellaneous Drugs					
Asparaginase	Elspar	IV	Acute lymphocytic leukemia	IV: 200 IU/kg daily for 28 days	Allergic reactions Pancreatitis
Cisplatin (CDDP)	Platinol	IV	Testicular tumor Ovarian carcinoma Head and neck cancer Lung cancer	IV: 100 mg/M^2 once every 4 weeks	Patients must be well hydrated prior to therapy Renal tubular damage Neurotoxicity Ototoxicity Myelosuppression
Etoposide	VePesid	PO: 50 mg cap IV	Testicular neoplasms Small cell lung cancer	Numerous schedules are used	Bone marrow depression Nausea, vomiting

Hydroxyurea	Hydrea	PO: 500 mg cap	Chronic myelogenous leukemia and others	PO: 20–30 mg/kg daily	Bone marrow depression
Interferon alfa	Alferon Intron Roferon	IM SQ	Chronic myelogenous leukemia Hairy cell leukemia AIDS-related Kaposi's sarcoma	Numerous schedules are used	Flu-like syndrome
Leuprolide	Lupron	IM SQ	Metastatic prostatic carcinoma	IM: 7.5 mg every month	Hot flashes
Procarbazine	Matulane	PO: 50 mg cap	Hodgkin's disease Brain and other tumors	PO: 100 mg/M^2 daily for 14 days each month (part of MOPP regimen)	Bone marrow depression
Tamoxifen	Nolvadex	PO: 10 mg tab	Breast cancer (estrogen-receptor positive)	PO: 10–20 mg twice daily	Nausea, vomiting, hot flashes

CARDIOVASCULAR DRUGS

Afterload-Reducing Agents
Afterload-reducing agents, or vasodilators, may be indicated for severe, low-output heart failure. Therapy must be individualized, and careful attention should be given to monitoring of the patient.

GENERIC NAME	TRADE NAME	PREPARATIONS	GENERAL INDICATIONS	USUAL DOSAGE	CAUTIONS / COMMENTS
Captopril	Capoten	PO: 12.5, 25, 50, 100 mg tab	Heart failure Also used for hypertension	PO: Initially 12.5 mg 3 times daily	Proteinuria Neutropenia Postural hypotension Hyperkalemia Cough
Enalapril	Vasotec	PO: 2.5, 5, 10, 20 mg tab	Heart failure Also used for hypertension	PO: 2.5–5 mg once daily and gradually increase to maintenance dose of 10–40 mg daily	Similar to captopril
Hydralazine	Apresoline	PO: 10, 25, 50, 100 mg tab	Heart failure	PO: 50 mg every 6 h	Headache, SLE syndrome, tachycardia, fluid retention
Isosorbide dinitrate	Isordil Sorbitrate Generic	PO: 2.5, 5, 10, 20, 40 mg timed-release tab	Heart failure	PO: 5–80 mg 3–4 times daily	Orthostatic hypotension, headache
Lisinopril	Prinivil Zestril	PO: 5, 10, 20, 40 mg tab	Heart failure Also used for hypertension	PO: Initially 10 mg once daily Usual dosage range is 20–40 mg/day	Similar to captopril
Nifedipine	Adalat Procardia	PO: 10, 20 mg cap	Heart failure Also used for hypertension and angina	PO: 10–30 mg every 8 h	Postural hypotension Peripheral edema Extended-release preparation available

Drug	Brand	Dosage Forms	Indications	Dosing	Comments
Nitroglycerin 2% ointment	Nitro-Bid Nitrol Nitrong Generic	Topical: 15 mg per inch	Heart failure	Topical: 1.5 to 4 inches on skin	Orthostatic hypotension, headache Effects last 3–6 h
Nitroprusside	Nipride	IV	Heart failure	IV: 0.5–10 μg/kg/min; start at low dose and gradually increase infusion	Useful for short-term therapy Direct arterial pressure monitoring is essential Hypotension is a possible adverse reaction
Prazosin	Minipress	PO: 0.5, 1, 2, 5 mg cap	Heart failure	PO: 1 mg 2–3 times daily initially Range: 6–15 mg daily	Orthostatic hypotension
Antianginal Agents					
Acebutolol	Sectral	PO: 200, 400 mg caps	Angina Also used for hypertension	PO: 200 mg twice daily, increase up to 1200 mg daily if necessary	Similar to propranolol
Atenolol	Tenormin	PO: 25, 50, 100 mg tab IV: 0.5 mg/ml	Angina Also used for hypertension	PO: 50 mg once daily, may increase to 100 mg daily	Similar to propranolol
Diltiazem	Cardizem	PO: 30, 60, 90, 120 mg tab	Angina, vasospastic angina, chronic angina	PO: 30 mg 4 times daily, may increase up to 90 mg 4 times daily	Use cautiously in combination with β-blocker, may worsen heart block Extended-release preparation available
Dipyridamole	Persantine	PO: 25 mg tab	Prophylaxis of angina	PO: 50 mg 3 times daily, taken at least 1 h before meals	Headache, dizziness, syncope, GI disturbances

Table continued on following page

GENERIC NAME	TRADE NAME	PREPARATIONS	GENERAL INDICATIONS	USUAL DOSAGE	CAUTIONS/ COMMENTS
Erythrityl tetranitrate	Cardilate	PO: 5, 10, 15 mg tab Sublingual	Prophylaxis of angina	For prophylaxis: PO: 10 mg 3 times daily For angina: sublingual 5 mg	
Isosorbide dinitrate	Isordil Sorbitrate Generic	PO: 2.5, 5, 10, 20 mg tab 40 mg timed-release cap and tab	Prophylaxis of angina Angina	For prophylaxis: PO: 5–80 mg 3–4 times daily For angina: sublingual 2.5–5 mg	
Metoprolol	Lopressor	PO: 50, 100 mg tab IV: 1 mg/ml	Angina Also used for hypertension	PO: 50 mg 2–4 times daily	Same as propranolol
Nadolol	Corgard	PO: 20, 40, 80, 120, 160 mg tab	Angina Also used for hypertension	PO: 40 mg initially once daily; increase by 40 mg every 3–7 days Usual range: 80–160 mg once daily	Similar to propranolol
Nifedipine	Adalat Procardia	PO: 10, 20 mg cap	Vasospastic angina, chronic angina Also used for arrhythmias	PO: 10–20 mg three times daily	Use cautiously in combination with β-blocker Extended-release preparation available
Nitroglycerin	Nitro-Bid Nitroglyn Nitrong Nitrospan (oral) Nitrostat (sublingual) Generic	PO: 2.5, 6.5, 9 mg tab and cap Sublingual 0.2, 0.3, 0.4, 0.6 mg tab	Angina Prophylaxis of angina	For angina: 0.4 mg sublingual; may repeat at 5-min intervals up to 3 times For prophylaxis: 2.5–6.5 mg 2–3 times daily	Headache, flushing, hypotension Old tablets lose potency

Drug	Brand	Preparation	Indication	Dosage	Comments
Nitroglycerin	Nitrostat	IV	Angina not responsive to other measures Also hypertension associated with MI	IV: 5 µg/min initially; titrate as needed	
Nitroglycerin 2% ointment	Nitro-Bid Nitrol Nitrong Generic	Ointment: 15 mg per inch	Angina	0.5–4 inches of paste every 4 h	Dosage must be individualized Effects last 3–6 h
Nitroglycerin patches	Nitrodisc Nitro-Dur Transderm-Nitro	Patches 2.5 mg/24 h (5 cm^2) 5 mg/24 h (10 cm^2) 10 mg/24 h (20 cm^2) 15 mg/24 h (30 cm^2)	Prophylaxis of angina	One patch daily	
Nitroglycerin spray	Nitrolingual spray	Metered dose: 0.4 mg per spray	Angina	One spray as needed repeat every 5 minutes	
Pindolol	Visken	PO: 5, 10 mg tab	Angina Also used for hypertension	PO: 10 mg 2 times daily; may increase up to 60 mg per day	Same as propranolol
Propranolol	Inderal	PO: 10, 20, 40, 80 mg tab; 80, 120, 160 long-acting cap; IV: 1 mg/ml	Angina Also used for tachycardia and hypertension (see other sections)	PO: 20–60 mg 3–4 times daily	May provoke bronchospasm, congestive heart failure Do not stop abruptly Extended-release preparation available
Timolol	Blocadren	PO: 5, 10, 20 mg tab	Angina	PO: 10–30 mg twice daily	Same as propranolol
Verapamil	Calan Isoptin	PO: 40, 80, 120 mg tab; IV: 2.5 mg/ml	Angina Vasospastic angina Also used for arrhythmias	PO: 80 mg 3–4 times daily; may increase to 480 mg total daily dose	Use cautiously in combination with β-blocker Extended-release preparation available

Table continued on following page

GENERIC NAME	TRADE NAME	PREPARATIONS	GENERAL INDICATIONS	USUAL DOSAGE	CAUTIONS / COMMENTS
Antiarrhythmics					
Adenosine	Adenocard	IV	Paroxysmal supraventricular tachycardia		
Amiodarone	Cordarone	PO	Life-threatening ventricular and supraventricular arrhythmias not responsive to other agents	PO: 200–600 mg daily	Requires oral loading dose during first month of therapy Pulmonary fibrosis Thyroid dysfunction Photosensitivity
Atropine		IV SC	Symptomatic bradycardia Heart block	IV, SC: 0.5–1.0 mg	Dry mouth Mydriasis
Bretylium	Bretylol	IV IM	Second drug of choice after lidocaine for ventricular fibrillation, ventricular tachycardia, or other ventricular arrhythmias	For ventricular fibrillation: IV: 5 mg/kg, may repeat in 15 min with 10 mg/kg Other ventricular arrhythmias: IV: 5–10 mg/kg diluted with 50 ml D5W over 10 min, may repeat every 6 h	For ventricular arrhythmias other than ventricular fibrillation, may also be given as constant infusion
Digoxin	Lanoxin Generic	IV PO: 0.125, 0.25, 0.5 mg tab	Rapid atrial fibrillation or atrial tachycardia	IV: 0.75 mg (dilute in 10 ml NS and give over 5–10 min) then 0.25–0.5 mg every 2–6 h × 1–3 PO: See under *Digitalis Preparations*	

Disopyramide	Norpace	PO: 100, 150 mg cap IV	Supraventricular tachyarrhythmias, ventricular arrhythmias, premature ventricular contractions	PO: 150 mg every 6 h IV: Loading dose 2 mg/kg over 15 min; may give additional 1–2 mg/kg over 45 min	Do not use in third degree block. May worsen CHF
Encainide	Enkaid	PO: 25, 35, 50 mg cap	Life-threatening ventricular arrhythmias	PO: 25–50 mg every 8–12 h	Dizziness, new or exacerbated arrhythmias Increased risk of sudden cardiac death in patients with underlying structural heart disease
Flecainide	Tambocor	PO: 100 mg tab	Ventricular and supraventricular arrhythmias not responsive to other agents	PO: 50 mg twice daily initially, usual maintenance 200–400 mg per day	Dizziness, CHF, new or exacerbated arrhythmias Increased risk of sudden cardiac death in patients with underlying structural heart disease
Isoproterenol	Isuprel	IV	Bradycardia and heart block unresponsive to atropine	IV: 1 mg diluted in 250 ml of D5W infused at rate of 1–10 μg/min	Can cause arrhythmias—use with caution in acute myocardial infarction
Lidocaine	Xylocaine	IV IM	Ventricular fibrillation, ventricular irritability, and ventricular tachycardia Prophylaxis following acute MI	IV: 50–100 mg over 2 min, then 1–4 mg/min IM: 300 mg	Do not use in third degree block Reduce dosage in patients with CHF and liver failure CNS side effects (twitching, agitation, convulsions, drowsiness) IM use as indicated when an IV cannot be started

Table continued on following page

GENERIC NAME	TRADE NAME	PREPARATIONS	GENERAL INDICATIONS	USUAL DOSAGE	CAUTIONS / COMMENTS
Mexiletine	Mexitil	PO: 150, 200, 250 mg cap	Ventricular arrhythmias	PO: Dosage must be individualized, usually 600–1200 mg daily in 3 divided doses	GI disturbances, dizziness, new or exacerbated arrhythmias
Phenytoin	Dilantin Generic	IV PO: 30, 100 mg cap	Digitalis toxicity and arrhythmias associated with tricyclic toxicity	IV: 50 mg every 2 min until control is achieved (not to exceed 1000 mg) PO: 1000 mg in first 24 h	Rapid IV administration may lead to hypotension Do not give IV with dextrose solutions
Procainamide	Pronestyl Procan SR Generic	IV IM PO: 250, 375, 500 mg cap and tab Sustained release (Procan SR): 250, 500 mg tab	Second drug of choice (after lidocaine) for ventricular irritability Oral use for supraventricular tachyarrhythmias and premature contractions	IV: 25–50 mg/min until controlled (loading dose not to exceed 1000 mg) followed by maintenance 1–4 mg/min PO: 250–500 mg every 3–4 h Sustained release: 500 mg–1 g every 6 h	Do not use in third degree block Side effects include nausea, vomiting, hypotension, widened QRS, arrhythmias May cause lupus-like syndrome
Propranolol	Inderal	IV PO: 10, 20, 40, 80 mg tab; 80, 120, 160 long-acting cap	Tachycardias Also used for angina and hypertension (see other sections)	IV: 0.5–1 mg/min up to 5 mg PO: 10–80 mg 3–4 times daily	Do not use in third degree block Depresses myocardial contractility and can cause bronchospasm in asthma patients

Drug	Trade Name	Preparation	Indications	Dosage	Comments
Quinidine gluconate	Duraquin Quinaglute	IV ⎱ rarely used IM ⎰ PO: Gluconate: 324, 330 mg tab (sustained release)	Supraventricular arrhythmias Premature contractions and maintenance after conversion from atrial fibrillation	324–972 mg every 8 h	Side effects include hypotension, widened QRS, nausea, diarrhea, ventricular arrhythmias
Quinidine sulfate	Quinidex Generic	Sulfate: 100, 200, 300 mg tab		200–400 mg every 6 h	
Tocainide	Tonocard	PO: 400, 600 mg tab	Ventricular arrhythmias	PO: 400 mg three times daily up to maximum of 2400 mg daily in divided doses	CNS side effects, GI side effects, rash
Verapamil	Isoptin Calan	IV: 2.5 mg/ml PO: 80, 120 mg tab	Atrial fibrillation, atrial flutter, paroxysmal supraventricular tachycardia Also used for angina (PO)	IV: 5 mg over 60 seconds (over 3 min in elderly patients); may repeat with 10 mg in 15 minutes	Hypotension
Anticlaudication Drugs					
Pentoxifylline	Trental	PO: 400 mg tab	Intermittent claudication	PO: 400 mg 3 times daily with meals	Nausea, dizziness, headache
Antihypertensives					
Acebutolol	Sectral	PO: 400 mg cap	Mild to moderate hypertension	PO: 400 mg once daily	
Atenolol	Tenormin	PO: 25, 50, 100 mg tab	Mild to moderate hypertension	PO: 50 mg daily; may increase to 100 mg daily	See propranolol Sustained-release preparation available
Captopril	Capoten	PO: 12.5, 25, 50, 100 mg tab	Moderate to severe hypertension	PO: 12.5–25 mg 3 times daily—dosage must be individualized up to 150 mg 3 times daily	Used with diuretic Proteinuria, neutropenia, postural hypotension, cough

Table continued on following page

215

GENERIC NAME	TRADE NAME	PREPARATIONS	GENERAL INDICATIONS	USUAL DOSAGE	CAUTIONS / COMMENTS
Clonidine	Catapres	PO: 0.1, 0.2 mg tab Patches: 3 sizes	Moderate hypertension	PO: 0.1 mg 2–3 times daily Usual maintenance dose is 0.2–0.8 mg daily Patches: once a week	Withdrawal reaction with abrupt discontinuation
Diazoxide	Hyperstat	IV	Hypertensive crisis	IV: 300 mg push, may repeat in 30 min	Should give furosemide IV to prevent fluid overload
Enalapril	Vasotec	PO: 2.5, 5, 10, 20 mg tab	Moderate to severe hypertension	PO: 2.5 mg initially; maintenance 10–40 mg daily	See *Captopril*
Enalaprilat		IV		IV: 1.25 mg q 6 h	
Guanabenz	Wytensin	PO: 4, 8 mg tab	Mild to moderate hypertension	PO: 4 mg twice daily; increase as needed up to 65 mg daily	Sedation, dryness of mouth
Guanethidine	Ismelin	PO: 10, 25 mg tab	Moderate to severe hypertension	PO: 10–25 mg daily	Postural hypotension is a frequent side effect
Hydralazine	Apresoline Generic	IV PO: 10, 25, 50, 100 mg tab	Hypertensive crisis Moderate to severe hypertension	IV: 10–20 mg slowly PO: 10–25 mg 2–3 times daily	May cause lupus-like syndrome
Labetalol	Trandate Normodyne	IV PO: 100, 200, 300, 400 mg tab	Severe hypertension Hypertensive crisis	IV: 20 mg slowly over 2 min; dosage must be individualized PO: 100 mg twice daily initially; 200–800 mg daily for moderate hypertension	GI disturbances Orthostatic hypotension
Lisinopril	Prinivil Zestril	PO: 10, 20, 40, 80 mg tab	Moderate to severe hypertension	PO: 10–80 mg once daily	See *Captopril*

Generic	Trade	Forms	Indications	Dosage	Comments
Methyldopa	Aldomet	IV PO: 125, 250, 500 mg tab	Mild to moderate hypertension	IV: 250–500 mg every 6–8 h PO: 250 mg once or twice daily	Drowsiness, depression Positive Coombs' test occurs with prolonged therapy in 20% of patients
Metoprolol	Lopressor	PO: 50, 100 mg tab	Moderate to severe hypertension	PO: 50 mg twice daily, increase as needed at weekly intervals (maximum 450 mg daily)	More β selective than propranolol Do not stop abruptly Can cause bronchospasm in patients with asthma and COPD
Minoxidil	Loniten	PO: 2.5, 10 mg tab	Severe refractory hypertension in patients with advanced renal disease	PO: 2.5 mg twice daily	Fluid retention, tachycardia, hypertrichosis Should be administered only by physicians familiar with its use
Nadolol	Corgard	PO: 40, 80, 120 mg tab	Moderate to severe hypertension Angina	PO: 40 mg once daily, may increase gradually by 40–80 mg increments every 3–7 days Usual maintenance dose is 80–320 mg/day	Do not use in third degree block Depresses myocardial contractility and can cause bronchospasm in asthma patients
Nifedipine	Procardia Adalat	PO: 10, 20 mg cap	Hypertensive crisis Hypertension	PO: 10 mg 3–4 times daily; may increase to maximum of 120–180 mg daily For crisis: sublingual—break 10 mg cap; may repeat in 20–30 min	Hypotension Peripheral edema Sustained-release preparation available

Table continued on following page

GENERIC NAME	TRADE NAME	PREPARATIONS	GENERAL INDICATIONS	USUAL DOSAGE	CAUTIONS / COMMENTS
Nitroprusside	Nipride	IV	Hypertensive crisis	IV: 0.5–10 µg/kg/min; start at low dose and titrate for effect	Should only be used in intensive care setting Protect solution from light Thiocyanate toxicity possible during prolonged infusion
Pindolol	Visken	PO: 5, 10 mg tab	Mild to moderate hypertension	PO: 10 mg twice daily; may increase to 60 mg daily	See propranolol
Prazosin	Minipress	PO: 1, 2, 5, mg cap	Moderate to severe hypertension	PO: 1 mg at bedtime; initially 1 mg 2–3 times daily, may increase up to 20 mg daily	Orthostatic hypotension at onset of therapy
Propranolol	Inderal Inderal LA	PO: 10, 20, 40, 80 mg tab Long-acting: 80, 120, 160 mg cap	Mild to moderate hypertension Also for angina and tachycardia (see other sections)	PO: 20–40 mg twice daily Long-acting: 80 mg daily	Do not stop abruptly May cause bronchospasm in patients with asthma or COPD
Reserpine	Serpasil Generic	PO: 0.1, 0.25 mg tab IM	Moderate hypertension Hypertensive emergencies	PO: 0.1–0.5 mg daily; dosage must be individualized IM: 0.5–1.0 mg followed by 2–4 mg at 3–12 h intervals	Nasal congestion, postural hypotension, male impotence, depression
Timolol	Blocadren	PO: 5, 10, 20 mg tab	Mild to moderate hypertension	PO: 10 mg twice daily initially; usually maintenance 20–40 mg daily	See propranolol

Digitalis Preparations

Digitoxin	Crystodigin Purodigin Generic	IV IM PO: 0.05, 0.1, 0.15, 0.2 mg tab	Congestive heart failure Rapid atrial fibrillation	For rapid oral digitalization: 0.8 mg initially, then 0.2 mg every 6–8 h for 2–3 doses Usual maintenance dose is 0.1 mg/day (0.05–0.2 mg)	Longer half-life than digoxin; therefore, toxicity is more difficult to manage
Digoxin	Lanoxin Generic	IV PO: 0.125, 0.25, 0.5 mg tab	Congestive heart failure Rapid atrial fibrillation (see under *Antiarrhythmics*)	For rapid IV digitalization: 0.25–0.5 mg followed by 0.25 mg every 4–6 h up to 1.5 mg For rapid oral digitalization: 0.5–0.75 mg followed by 0.25–0.5 mg every 6–8 h until full digitalization (usually 1.5 mg) Usual maintenance dose is 0.125–0.375 mg/day	Decrease maintenance dosage with renal impairment and in elderly patients
Ouabain	Generic	IV	Pulmonary edema Rapid atrial fibrillation	IV: 0.25–0.5 mg initially, then 0.1 mg every h (maximum 1 mg/24 h)	Rapid-acting, used in emergencies

Diuretics

Thiazides (or related agents) or more potent diuretics are usually a part of antihypertensive regimens

Chlorothiazide	Diuril Generic	IV PO: 250, 500 mg tab		IV: 500 mg twice daily PO: 250–500 mg once or twice daily	Hypokalemia Duration of action: 6–12 h

Table continued on following page

GENERIC NAME	TRADE NAME	PREPARATIONS	GENERAL INDICATIONS	USUAL DOSAGE	CAUTIONS / COMMENTS
Cyclothiazide	Anhydron	PO: 2 mg tab		PO: 2 mg once daily	Hypokalemia Duration of action: 18–24 h
Hydrochlorothiazide	HydroDiuril Esidrix Oretic Generic	PO: 25, 50 mg tab		PO: 25–50 mg once or twice daily	Hypokalemia Duration of action: 6–12 h
Indapamide	Lozol	PO: 2.5 mg tab		PO: 2.5 mg once daily	Hypokalemia
Trichlormethiazide	Naqua Metahydrin Generic	PO: 2, 4 mg tab		PO: 2–4 mg once daily	Hypokalemia Duration of action: 24 h
Other thiazide preparations are available					
Agents Related to Thiazides					
Chlorthalidone	Hygroton	PO: 25, 50, 100 mg tab		PO: 25–200 mg daily	Hypokalemia Duration of action: 24–72 h
Metolazone	Zaroxolyn Diulo	PO: 2.5, 5, 10 mg tab		PO: 2.5–5 mg daily	Hypokalemia Duration of action: 12–24 h
Loop Diuretics					
Bumetanide	Bumex	IV PO: 0.5, 1.0 mg		IV: 0.5–1.0 mg PO: 0.5–2.0 mg every other day	Hypokalemia Volume depletion
Ethacrynic acid	Edecrin	IV PO: 25, 50 mg tab		IV: 50 mg PO: 50–100 mg twice daily	Hypokalemia Volume depletion, hypochloremic alkalosis

Generic	Brand	Preparation	Indication	Dosage	Comments
Furosemide	Lasix	IV PO: 20, 40, 80 mg tab		IV: 20–40 mg PO: 20–40 mg twice daily	Hypokalemia Volume depletion, hypochloremic alkalosis

Potassium-Sparing Diuretics. May be used in combination with thiazide to prevent hypokalemia

Generic	Brand	Preparation	Indication	Dosage	Comments
Amiloride	Midamor	PO: 5 mg		PO: 5–10 mg daily	Hyperkalemia
Spironolactone	Aldactone	PO: 25 mg tab		PO: 25–50 mg twice daily	Hyperkalemia Use with caution in patients with renal failure
Triamterene	Dyrenium	PO: 50, 100 mg cap		PO: 100 mg twice daily (after a week, maximum 300 mg/day)	Hyperkalemia Use with caution in patients with renal failure

Combination Thiazide and Potassium-Sparing Diuretics

Generic	Brand	Preparation	Indication	Dosage	Comments
Amiloride, hydrochlorothiazide	Moduretic	PO: Tab, contains 5 mg amiloride and 50 mg hydrochlorothiazide		PO: 1–2 tab daily	Monitoring of serum K^+ is still important
Spironolactone, hydrochlorothiazide	Aldactazide	PO: Tab, contains 25 mg of each		PO: 1–2 tab twice daily	Monitoring of serum K^+ is still important
Triamterene, hydrochlorothiazide	Dyazide	PO: Cap, contains 50 mg triamterene and 25 mg hydrochlorothiazide		PO: 1–2 cap twice daily	Monitoring of serum K^+ is still important

Intravenous Vasoactive Drugs

Generic	Brand	Preparation	Indication	Dosage	Comments
Amrinone	Inocor	IV	Short-term therapy for severe congestive heart failure refractory to other drugs	IV: 0.75 mg/kg IV over 2–3 min followed by infusion of 5–10 µg/kg/min	Hypotension, fever, vomiting, diarrhea Avoid with disopyramide
Dobutamine	Dobutrex	IV	Short term therapy to increase cardiac output	IV: 2.5–10 µg/kg/min	Tachycardia, increased rate in patient in atrial fibrillation

Table continued on following page

GENERIC NAME	TRADE NAME	PREPARATIONS	GENERAL INDICATIONS	USUAL DOSAGE	CAUTIONS/COMMENTS
Dopamine	Intropin Dopastat	IV	Cardiogenic and septic shock	IV: 200 mg in 250 ml D5W (800 μg/ml) Infuse at slow rate of 2–5 μg/kg/min and increase up to 50 μg/kg/min until effect is achieved	GI side effects CNS stimulation, tachyarrhythmias Oliguria at higher doses At lower doses may increase renal and mesenteric blood flow
Epinephrine	Adrenalin	IV SC	Asystole, refractory VF Anaphylactic shock	For asystole: 10 ml of 1:10,000 IV, intracardiac, or by endotracheal tube For anaphylaxis: 0.5 ml of 1:1000 SC or IV (if shock is present)	Tachycardia, atrial and ventricular arrhythmias, anxiety
Isoproterenol	Isuprel	IV	Bradycardia Torsades de pointes	IV: 1 mg in 500 ml D5W (2 μg/ml) Infuse at 1–10 μg/min	Arrhythmias may occur Possible hypotension
Levarterenol (norepinephrine)	Levophed	IV	Cardiogenic shock	IV: 4–8 mg in 500 ml D5W and titrated for effect (start at 8 μg/min)	Tissue necrosis with extravasation
Metaraminol	Aramine	IV IM	Shock	IM: 5–10 mg IV: 200–500 mg diluted in 1000 ml D5W and titrated for effect	IV route is preferred
Phenylephrine	Neo-Synephrine	IV IM	Shock	IM: 1–10 mg IV: 0.04–0.18 mg/min, titrated for effect	IV route is preferred End-organ ischemia

DERMATOLOGIC DRUGS

GENERIC NAME	TRADE NAME	PREPARATIONS	USUAL DOSAGE	GENERAL INDICATIONS	CAUTIONS / COMMENTS
Topical Steroids		Many topical steroids in varying strengths are available, and the following table lists a selection based on potency. Group 1 is the most potent and Group 7 the least potent. All except the weakest preparations can suppress adrenal function when used under occlusive dressing.			
Group 1 Betamethasone in optimized vehicle	Diprolene	Cream and ointment 0.05%			Extremely potent—can have effect on adrenal function
Clobetasol	Temovate	Cream and ointment 0.05%			Extremely potent
Group 2 Amcinonide	Cyclocort	Ointment 0.1%			
Betamethasone	Diprosone	Ointment 0.05%			
Desoximetasone	Topicort	Cream 0.25% Ointment 0.25%			
Diflorasone	Florone Maxiflor	Ointment 0.5% Ointment 0.05%			
Fluocinonide	Lidex	Cream 0.05% Gel 0.05% Ointment 0.05%			
Halcinonide	Halog	Cream 0.1%			
Group 3 Betamethasone	Diprosone Valisone	Cream 0.05% Ointment 0.1%			

Table continued on following page

223

GENERIC NAME	TRADE NAME	PREPARATIONS	GENERAL INDICATIONS	USUAL DOSAGE	CAUTIONS / COMMENTS
Diflorasone	Florone Maxiflor	Cream 0.05% Cream 0.05%			
Triamcinolone	Aristocort	Cream (HP) 0.5%			
Group 4 Betamethasone Desoximetasone	Benisone Topicort LP	Ointment 0.025% Cream 0.05%			
Fluocinolone	Synalar	Cream (HP) 0.2% Ointment 0.05%			
Flurandrenolide	Cordran	Ointment 0.05%			
Triamcinolone	Aristocort Kenalog	Ointment 0.025% Ointment 0.1%			
Group 5 Betamethasone	Diprosone Valisone	Lotion 0.02% Cream 0.1% Lotion 0.1%			
Fluocinolone	Synalar	Cream 0.1%			
Flurandrenolide	Cordran	Cream 0.05%			
Hydrocortisone butyrate	Locoid	Cream 0.1% Ointment 0.1%			
Hydrocortisone valerate	Westcort	Cream 0.2%			
Trimacinolone	Kenalog	Cream 0.1% Lotion 0.1%			

Group 6				
Desonide	DesOwen Tridesilon	Cream 0.05% Cream 0.05%		
Flumethasone	Locorten	Cream 0.03%		
Fluocinolone	Synalar	Solution 0.01%		
Group 7				
Hydrocortisone	Generic Generic	Cream ½% OTC, 1%, 2.5% Lotion 1%, 2.5% Ointment 1%, 2.5%		
Miscellaneous Drugs				
Aluminum acetate (Burow's solution)	Bluboro Domeboro Generic	Topical solution, tablets or powder Dilute 30 ml stock solution in 1–2 liters of tepid or cool water or one tablet or packet in 1 liter of water	Cleansing and débriding to dry exudative lesions	Apply using compresses as needed	Use "open" compress technique, which allows evaporation and cooling
Benzoyl peroxide	Benoxyl Benzagel Desquam-X Persadox Others Generic	Topical: 5%, 10% lotion 5% cream	Acne	Apply to involved area once or twice daily	
Podophyllin	Podoben Generic	Topical: 25% in tincture of benzoin	Condylomata acuminata	Apply to involved area; wash off 4 h later	Avoid contact with normal skin; may protect with petrolatum Excessive use may be toxic Avoid in pregnancy

Table continued on following page

GENERIC NAME	TRADE NAME	PREPARATIONS	GENERAL INDICATIONS	USUAL DOSAGE	CAUTIONS / COMMENTS
Selenium sulfide	Selsun Selsun Blue Exsel Generic	Topical: 2.5% suspension 2.5% lotion 1% cream, lotion, or shampoo	Dandruff Tinea versicolor	Apply 1–2 tsp to scalp or affected area and wash off after 2–3 minutes	2.5% suspension requires prescription
Tretinoin	Retin-A	Topical: 0.05%, 0.1% cream 0.025% gel (Retin-A)	Acne	Apply to involved areas daily	Local irritation—should not be used if other drying agents are used Avoid mucous membrane

ENDOCRINE DRUGS

GENERIC NAME	TRADE NAME	PREPARATIONS	GENERAL INDICATIONS	USUAL DOSAGE	CAUTIONS/COMMENTS
Hypoglycemic Agents, Oral					
		All of the sulfonylurea compounds can cause hypoglycemia. The possibility that sulfonylureas may be associated with adverse cardiac outcomes remains a controversial issue.			
First Generation Sulfonylureas					
Acetohexamide	Dymelor	PO: 250, 500 mg tab	Type II diabetes not responsive to diet	Should be individualized Range: 250 mg–1.5 g daily	Doses under 1 g can be given as daily dose; larger daily doses should be divided Use cautiously in elderly patients and in renal insufficiency
Chlorpropamide	Diabinese	PO: 100, 250 mg tab	Type II diabetes not responsive to diet	Should be individualized 100–500 mg daily at breakfast	Long acting Can cause hyponatremia or flushing
Tolazamide	Tolinase	PO: 100, 250, 500 mg tab	Type II diabetes not responsive to diet	Should be individualized Initially, 100–250 mg daily at breakfast Adjust every 4–6 days until a maintenance dose is reached (maximum 1 g)	Daily doses of 500 mg or greater should be divided
Tolbutamide	Orinase	PO: 500 mg tab	Type II diabetes not responsive to diet	Should be individualized Initially, 500 mg b.i.d., adjusted as necessary Usual maintenance dose: 250 mg–3g daily in single or divided doses	Shorter duration than other oral agents

Table continued on following page

GENERIC NAME	TRADE NAME	PREPARATIONS	GENERAL INDICATIONS	USUAL DOSAGE	CAUTIONS/COMMENTS
Second Generation Sulfonylureas					
Glyburide	DiaBeta Micronase	PO: 1.25, 2.5, 5 mg tab	Type II diabetes not responsive to diet	PO: 5 mg daily initially Dosage should be individualized Range: 1.25–30 mg daily	Caution in patients with renal insufficiency
Glipizide	Glucotrol	PO: 5, 10 mg tab	Type II diabetes not responsive to diet	PO: 5 mg daily initially Dosage should be individualized Range: 2.5–40 mg daily	

Hypoglycemic Agents, Parenteral—Insulin Preparations

Rapid-Acting Preparations

TYPE	ONSET	MAXIMAL EFFECT	DURATION	PREPARATIONS
Regular	½–1 h	2–3 h	5–8 h	Pork Beef Beef-pork Human semisynthetic Human recombinant DNA
Zinc suspension, Semilente Insulin	½–3 h	4–6 h	12–16 h	Pork Beef Beef-pork

Intermediate-Acting Preparations

NPH	1–1½ h	8–12 h	16–24 h	Pork Beef Beef-pork Human semisynthetic Human recombinant DNA
Zinc suspension, Lente Insulin	1–3 h	8–12 h	18–28 h	Pork Beef Beef-pork Human semisynthetic Human recombinant DNA

Long-Acting Preparations

Zinc suspension, Ultralente Insulin	4–8 h	16–18 h	36+ h	Beef Beef-pork
Protamine, Zinc	4–8 h	16–18 h	36+ h	Pork Beef Beef-pork

GENERIC NAME	TRADE NAME	PREPARATIONS	GENERAL INDICATIONS	USUAL DOSAGE	CAUTIONS/COMMENTS
Lipid-Lowering Agents Cholestyramine resin	Questran	PO: Packets (9 g) contain 4 g of active drug—mix in 4–6 oz of suitable liquid	Increased LDL cholesterol (high cholesterol and normal triglyceride)	4 g (one packet) 4 times daily, may increase to 6 g 4 times daily	Bloating, mild nausea, and constipation Malabsorption may be noted at doses > 30 g/day

Table continued on following page

GENERIC NAME	TRADE NAME	PREPARATIONS	GENERAL INDICATIONS	USUAL DOSAGE	CAUTIONS/COMMENTS
Clofibrate	Atromid-S	PO: 500 mg cap	Increased VLDL levels	500 mg 2–4 times daily	GI side effects Increased incidence of cholelithiasis Clofibrate interferes with Coumadin and phenytoin Contraindicated in patients with renal or hepatic failure Use cautiously in patients with ischemic heart disease Possible association with GI malignancies
Colestipol	Colestid	PO: Packets (5 g)	Same as cholestyramine	PO: 15–30 g daily divided in 2–4 doses with meals	Same as cholestyramine
Gemfibrozil	Lopid	PO: 300 mg cap	Same as clofibrate	PO: 600 mg 30 min before breakfast and dinner	GI side effects, increases HDL levels
Lovastatin	Mevacor	PO: 10, 20, 40 mg tab	Increased LDL cholesterol	10–80 mg/day divided into 1–2 doses	Possible GI side effects Elevated hepatic transaminases Rare myositis and myopathy
Niacin (Nicotinic acid)	Nicolar Nicobid Generic	PO: 500 mg tab	Severe hypertriglyceridemia With bile acid resins, used for familial hypercholesterolemia	Initially, low dose of 100 mg 3 times daily Increase gradually to maintenance dose of 1.5–6 g daily (in divided doses)	Flushing Pruritus GI side effects (peptic ulcer flare-up) Hyperuricemia Liver dysfunction Exacerbation of diabetes

Drug	Brand	Form/Dose	Indication	Dosing	Comments
Probucol	Lorelco	PO: 250 mg tab	Increases LDL levels Best used in combination with bile acid resins or niacin	PO: 500 mg twice daily with meals	GI disturbances Decreases HDL levels

Osteoporotic Agents
Calcium Preparations

Drug	Brand	Form/Dose	Indication	Dosing	Comments
Milk		All forms: 300 mg/8 oz elemental calcium	Prevention of negative calcium balance	1500 mg elemental calcium daily is felt to be the optimal dose	Lactase deficiency or malabsorption may require use of supplements or yogurt
Cheese		Solid—200 mg/oz elemental calcium Cottage—200 mg/8 oz elemental calcium		To achieve a 1500 mg daily dose, a combination of calcium preparations and dairy products can be used	May be high in fat and sodium content
Calcium carbonate	Tums	500 mg (200 mg elemental calcium)		6–8 tab daily	Caution if at risk for nephrolithiasis
Calcium (oyster shell)	Os-Cal Others	500 mg (250 mg elemental calcium)		6 tab daily	
Calcium lactate		650 mg (87 mg elemental calcium)		17 tab daily	
Calcium gluconate		1000 mg (90–100 mg elemental calcium)		15 tab daily	

Estrogens

Drug	Brand	Form/Dose	Indication	Dosing	Comments
Estrogens, conjugated	Premarin	0.3 mg, 0.625 mg, 1.25 mg, 2.5 mg	Post menopausal females at risk for osteoporosis	0.625 mg daily for 3 weeks out of every 4	Usual contraindications for estrogen therapy Cyclic therapy with progestinal agent usually recommended if uterus still present

Table continued on following page

GENERIC NAME	TRADE NAME	PREPARATIONS	GENERAL INDICATIONS	USUAL DOSAGE	CAUTIONS/COMMENTS
Ethinyl estradiol	Many names	Multiple		25 μg daily for 3 weeks out of every 4	
Medroxy-progesterone acetate	Provera			10 mg daily for the last 7–10 days of the month, at least every 3rd month	Must obtain PAP smear q 6–18 months
Vitamin D	Generic	Vitamin D Vitamin D_2 Vitamin D_3	Vitamin D deficiency	Vitamin D deficiency: 50,000 units daily for 1–3 months	Must monitor serum and urinary calcium
			May be indicated in patients without sun exposure	Lack of sun exposure, 50,000 units/week	Consultation with endocrinologist is recommended prior to use of high-dose Vitamin D
			Patients receiving pharmacologic doses of phenytoin, phenobarbitol, or corticosteroids	Chronic steroid therapy: 50,000 units/3 times weekly	
Steroids		Oral and parenteral steroids are discussed in this section. (See *Dermatologic Drugs* for topical steroid preparations.) The side effects associated with systemic steroid use, particularly longterm use, are numerous, and physicians should be acquainted with the potential risks prior to prescribing these drugs.			
Betamethasone	Celestone	IM Intraarticular Soft tissue PO: 0.6 mg tab	As antiinflammatory drug and for steroid replacement	IM: Must be individualized Intraarticular: 0.25–2.0 ml (1.5–12 mg) Soft tissue: 0.25–1 ml (0.25–6 mg)	Long-acting

Generic name	Trade names	Use	Route / Forms	Dosage	Comments
Cortisone	Cortone Generic	As antiinflammatory drug and for steroid replacement	IM PO: 5, 10, 25 mg tab	PO: Must be individualized Range: 0.6–7.2 mg daily IM: Must be individualized PO: Must be individualized Range: 25–150 mg daily	
Dexamethasone	Decadron Hexadrol Generic	As antiinflammatory drug and for steroid replacement Used for cerebral edema	IV IM Intraarticular Soft tissue PO: 0.25, 0.5, 0.75, 1.5, 4 mg tab	IV, IM: Must be individualized Intraarticular: 0.5–2 ml (4–16 mg) Soft tissue: 0.5–2 ml (4–16 mg) PO: Must be individualized Range: 0.75–9 mg daily in 2–4 doses	Long-acting
Fludrocortisone	Florinef	Replacement therapy for mineralocorticoid insufficiency	PO: 0.1 mg tab	PO: 0.1 mg daily	For adrenal insufficiency, should be combined with a glucocorticoid
Hydrocortisone* (cortisol)	Cortef Solu-Cortef Others Generic	As antiinflammatory drug and for steroid replacement	IV IM Intraarticular Soft tissue Rectal: 100 mg enemas PO: 5, 10, 20 mg tab	IV: 100–500 mg IM: To be used only if IV route not possible—100–250 mg Intraarticular: 5–50 mg Soft tissue: 25–75 mg PO: Must be individualized Range: 10–240 mg daily	Short-acting

Table continued on following page

GENERIC NAME	TRADE NAME	PREPARATIONS	GENERAL INDICATIONS	USUAL DOSAGE	CAUTIONS/COMMENTS
Methylprednisolone*	Medrol Solu-Medrol Depo-Medrol Generic	IV IM Intraarticular Soft tissue PO: 2, 4, 8, 16, 24, 32 mg tab	As antiinflammatory drug and for steroid replacement	IV, IM: Must be individualized Intraarticular: 4–80 mg Soft tissue: 10–40 mg PO: Must be individualized Range: 4–16 mg daily	
Prednisolone	Delta-Cortef Sterane Others Generic	IV IM Intraarticular Soft tissue PO: 1, 2.5, 5 mg tab	As antiinflammatory drug and for steroid replacement	IV, IM: 20–100 mg Intraarticular: 4–30 mg Soft tissue: 8–60 mg PO: Must be individualized Range: 5–60 mg daily	
Prednisone	Deltasone Meticorten Orasone Generic	PO: 1, 2.5, 5, 10, 20, 50 mg tab	As antiinflammatory drug and for steroid replacement	Must be individualized Range: 5–60 mg daily	
Triamcinolone	Aristocort Kenacort Others Generic	IM Intraarticular Soft tissue PO: 1, 2, 4, 8, 15 mg tab	As antiinflammatory drug and for steroid replacement	IM: 40 mg Intraarticular: 2.5–80 mg Soft tissue: 5–40 mg PO: Must be individualized Range: 4–40 mg	Long-acting

*See table on page 238 for potency and activity.

GENERIC NAME	TRADE NAME	PREPARATIONS	GENERAL INDICATIONS	USUAL DOSAGE	CAUTIONS/COMMENTS
Thyroid Preparations					
Hyperthyroid Agents					
Methimazole	Tapazole	PO: 5, 10 mg tab	Hyperthyroidism and thyrotoxic crisis	For hyperthyroidism: 15–60 mg initially daily in 4 doses Maintenance dose: 10–30 mg daily in 2–3 doses	Agranulocytosis Rash
Potassium iodide	Lugol's solution Generic (SSKI)	IV PO	Thyrotoxic crisis Preparation for thyroidectomy	For thyrotoxic crisis: IV: 250–500 mg daily, or sodium iodide 1 g every 8 h PO: SSKI 10 drops 3 times daily For preparation for surgery: PO: 2–6 drops Lugol's solution 3 times daily for 10 days	
Propranolol (and other β-blockers)	Inderal	IV PO: 10, 20, 40, 80 mg tab	Control of symptoms associated with hyperthyroidism	PO: 10–40 mg 4 times daily For symptoms associated with storm, thyrotoxic crisis: IV: 5 mg (slowly 1 mg/min) Total dose 2–10 mg every 3–4 h PO: 20–160 mg every 4–8 h	Relative contraindications: CHF, asthma

Table continued on following page

GENERIC NAME	TRADE NAME	PREPARATIONS	GENERAL INDICATIONS	USUAL DOSAGE	CAUTIONS/COMMENTS
Propylthiouracil	Generic	PO: 50 mg tab	Hyperthyroidism and thyrotoxic crisis	For hyperthyroidism: PO: 300–600 mg daily in 3–4 doses initially Maintenance dose: 100–300 mg daily in 3 doses	Agranulocytosis Rash Pruritus
Hypothyroid Agents Levothyroxine	Synthroid Levothroid	IV PO: 0.025, 0.05, 0.1, 0.15, 0.175, 0.2, 0.3 mg tab	Myxedema coma Hypothyroidism	For myxedema: IV: 0.2 mg For hypothyroidism: PO: Usual maintenance dose—0.1–0.2 mg daily	Initiate PO therapy at lower dose and increase gradually Use cautiously in patients with ischemic heart disease
Liothyronine	Cytomel	IV PO: 5, 25, 50 µg tab	Hypothyroidism Myxedema coma	For myxedema: IV: 10–25 µg at 8–12 h intervals For hypothyroidism: PO: Usual maintenance dose—up to 75–100 µg daily	Initiate PO therapy at lower dose and increase gradually Use cautiously in patients with ischemic heart disease or arrhythmia
Liotrix	Euthroid Thyrolar	PO: Tabs, contain a mixture of levothyroxine and liothyronine in a 4:1 ratio Euthroid ½, 1, 2, and 3-grain tabs contain 30, 60,	Hypothyroidism	PO: Initially, Euthroid—½ or Thyrolar—½ daily Depending on response, dose is increased every 2 weeks	

120, and 180 μg of levothyroxine, respectively, and 7.5, 15, 30, and 45 μg of liothyronine, respectively

Thyrolar ¼-, ½-, 1-, 2-, 3-, and 5-grain tabs contain 12.5, 25, 50, 100, 150, and 250 μg of levothyronine, respectively, and 3.1, 6.25, 12.5, 25, 37.5, and 62.5 μg of liothyronine, respectively

Miscellaneous Drugs

Bromocriptine mesylate	Parlodel	PO: 2.5 mg, 5.0 mg	Persistent elevation of prolactin levels due to pituitary tumor	2.5–7.5 mg daily in divided doses	Very few side effects at low doses

GLUCOCORTICOID POTENCY AND MINERALOCORTICOID ACTIVITY OF SYSTEMIC STEROIDS*

Drug	Glucocorticoid Potency Compared with Hydrocortisone	Mineralocorticoid Activity
Hydrocortisone (cortisol)	1	+ +
Betamethasone	30	0
Cortisone	0.8	+ +
Dexamethasone	30	+
Fludrocortisone	0	+ + + +
Methylprednisolone	5	0
Prednisolone	4	+
Prednisone	4	+
Triamcinolone	5	0

*Adapted from AMA Drug Evaluations, 4th edition, Chicago, AMA, 1980, p. 620.

GASTROINTESTINAL DRUGS

GENERIC NAME	TRADE NAME	PREPARATIONS	COMMENTS
Antacids*			
Aluminum hydroxide	Amphojel AlternaGel Alu-Cap Alu-Tab	Tablets, capsules, and liquids	Constipating
Aluminum hydroxide, magnesium hydroxide	Maalox Mylanta Riopan	Tablets and liquid	Tend to cause diarrhea Riopan is low in sodium content Mylanta and Maalox Plus contain simethicone
Aluminum hydroxide, magnesium hydroxide, magnesium trisilicate	Gelusil-M	Tablets and liquid	Tends to cause diarrhea
Aluminum hydroxide, magnesium trisilicate	Gelusil	Tablets and liquid	Tends to cause diarrhea

*Antacids consist generally of aluminum hydroxide or trisilicate, calcium carbonate, or a combination. Dosage is 15–30 ml or 1–2 tablets as frequently as every hour. Numerous other antacid preparations are available

GENERIC NAME	TRADE NAME	PREPARATIONS	GENERAL INDICATIONS	USUAL DOSAGE	CAUTIONS/COMMENTS
Anticholinergics/Antispasmodics					
		A variety of anticholinergic preparations are available. They may be useful as adjuncts in treating patients with peptic ulcer disease whose pain is not relieved with antacids or by antiulcer drugs. Enough of the drug should be given to produce symptoms of dry mouth and blurred vision. These preparations are contraindicated in patients with heart disease, reflux esophagitis, pyloric obstruction, and urinary obstruction.			
Atropine		PO: 0.3, 0.4, 0.6 mg tab	Pain of peptic ulcer disease	PO: 0.3 to 1.2 mg every 4–6 h	The following are applicable to all anticholinergics/antispasmodics: Tachycardia Urinary hesitancy Nausea Constipation
Belladonna extract		PO: 15 mg tab	Pain of peptic ulcer disease	PO: 15 mg 3 times daily	
Belladonna tincture		PO: Liquid	Pain of peptic ulcer disease	PO: 1 ml 3–4 times daily	
Dicyclomine hydrochloride	Bentyl Dyspas Generic	PO: 10, 20 mg tab 10 mg cap	Pain of peptic ulcer disease	PO: 20 mg 3 times daily and 40 mg at bedtime	
Glycopyrrolate	Robinul Generic	PO: 1, 2 mg tab	Pain of peptic ulcer disease	PO: 1 mg 3 times daily and 2 mg at bedtime	
Propantheline bromide	Pro-Banthine Generic	PO: 7.5, 15 mg tab 30 mg timed-release tabs	Pain of peptic ulcer disease	PO: 15 mg 3 times daily and 30 mg at bedtime	
Antidiarrheal Drugs					
Bismuth subsalicylate	Pepto-Bismol	PO: Liquid	Diarrhea	PO: 30 ml up to 8 doses per day	Prophylaxis for traveler's diarrhea (60 ml q.i.d.) May discolor stool gray-black
Codeine		PO: 15, 30, 60 mg tab	Diarrhea	PO: 15–60 mg every 4–8 h	Prolonged use may lead to physical dependence

Drug	Trade name	Preparations	Indications	Dosage	Comments
Diphenoxylate	Lomotil	PO: Tab, contains 2.5 mg diphenoxylate and 0.025 mg atropine	Diarrhea	PO: 2 tabs up to 4 times daily	
Kaolin, pectin	Kaopectate Pargel	PO: Liquid	Diarrhea	PO: 2 ounces (60 ml) after each diarrheal stool	
Loperamide	Imodium	PO: 2 mg cap	Diarrhea	PO: 2 mg after each liquid stool (up to 16 mg/day)	
Opium tincture		PO: Liquid 10% contains 10 mg of morphine per ml	Diarrhea	PO: 1 ml every 4 h (up to 6 ml/day)	Prolonged use may lead to physical dependence
Paregoric (Camphorated tincture of opium)		PO: Liquid, contains 0.4 mg morphine per ml	Diarrhea	PO: 1–2 tsp up to 4 times daily	Prolonged use may lead to physical dependence
Antiemetics					
Cyclizine	Marezine	IM PO: 50 mg tab Suppository: 50, 100 mg	Postoperative nausea Motion sickness	IM, PO: 50 mg every 4–6 h Suppository: 100 mg 3–4 times daily	Drowsiness Dry mouth
Dimenhydrinate	Dramamine Generic	IV IM PO: 50 mg Suppository: 100 mg	Postoperative nausea Nausea and vomiting of pregnancy Motion sickness	IV, IM: 50 mg every 4 h PO: 50–100 mg every 4 h Suppository: 100 mg twice daily	Drowsiness
Diphenydramine	Benadryl Generic	IV IM PO: 25, 50 mg cap	Postoperative nausea Nausea of pregnancy Motion sickness	IV, IM: 10–20 mg every 2–3 h PO: 50 mg every 6 h	Drowsiness 25 mg available OTC

Table continued on following page

GENERIC NAME	TRADE NAME	PREPARATIONS	GENERAL INDICATIONS	USUAL DOSAGE	CAUTIONS/COMMENTS
Hydroxyzine	Atarax Marax Vistaril Generic	PO: 10, 25, 50, 100 mg tab and cap Solution available IM	Nausea and vomiting Pruritius, urticaria Anxiety	PO: 10–100 mg every 6 h IM: 25–100 mg every 6 h	Drowziness
Metoclopramide	Reglan	PO: 5, 10 mg tab Solution available IM IV	Nausea and vomiting Postoperative nausea	PO: 10 mg every 6 h IM: 10 mg every 4–6 h IV: 1–2 mg/kg every 2–3 h	IV route preferred for prevention of cancer chemotherapy-induced emesis Extrapyramidal reactions Diarrhea
Prochlorperazine	Compazine	IM PO: 5, 10 tab Suppository: 2.5, 5, 25 mg	Nausea and vomiting Postoperative nausea	IM, PO: 5–10 mg 3–4 times daily Suppository: 25 mg 2 times daily	Extrapyramidal reactions may occur, especially at higher dosages Not of benefit in motion sickness
Promethazine	Phenergan Remsed	IM PO: 25, 50, mg tab Suppository: 25, 50 mg	Postoperative nausea Motion sickness	IM, PO: 25 mg every 4–6 h Suppository: 25 mg every 4–6 h	
Scopolamine	Transderm-Scop	Transdermal 0.5 mg	Motion sickness	One patch for 3 days	Slight dry mouth
Trimethobenzamide	Tigan	IM PO: 100, 250 mg cap Suppository: 100, 200 mg	Nausea and vomiting Postoperative nausea	IM: 200 mg 3–5 times daily PO: 250 mg 3–4 times daily Suppository: 200 mg 3–4 times daily	Not of benefit in motion sickness

Antiinflammatory Bowel Drugs

Hydrocortisone enema	Cortenema	Enema: 100 mg	Ulcerative colitis, proctitis	Enema: once or twice daily
Mesalamine	Rowasa	Enema: 4 g Suppository: 500 mg	Ulcerative colitis, proctitis	Enema: once daily Suppository: 500 mg twice daily	Fewer side effects than oral sulfasalazine
Sulfasalazine	Azulfidine	PO: 500 mg tab Enema: 3 g	Ulcerative colitis	PO: 1–2 g 4 times daily	GI disturbances, blood dyscrasias

Antiulcer Drugs

Cimetidine	Tagamet	IV IM PO: 200, 300, 400 mg tab	Peptic ulcer disease	IV: 1–4 mg/kg/h or 300 mg over 1.5 min every 6 h IV: 300 mg every 6 h PO: 200, 300, 400 mg 4 times daily (with meals and at bedtime)	Depression, confusion Psychiatric side effects, especially in elderly
Famotidine	Pepcid	PO: 20, 40 mg tab Suspension available IV	Peptic ulcer disease	PO: 40 mg daily at bedtime IV: 20 mg every 12 h	Fewer CNS side effects than cimetidine
Misoprostol	Cytotec	PO: 100, 200 µg tab	Prevention of NSAID-induced ulcer	PO: 100–200 µg every 6 h	Diarrhea, abdominal pain Possible abortifacient effects
Ranitidine	Zantac	IV PO: 150, 300 mg tab	Peptic ulcer disease	IV: 75 to 150 mg IV every 12 h, or 6.25 mg/h by continuous infusion PO: 150 mg twice daily or 300 mg daily	Headache
Sucralfate	Carafate	PO: 1 g tab	Peptic ulcer disease	PO: 1 g 4 times daily 1 hour before meals or at bedtime	Constipation

Table continued on following page

243

GENERIC NAME	TRADE NAME	PREPARATIONS	GENERAL INDICATIONS	USUAL DOSAGE	CAUTIONS/COMMENTS
Gastroparetic Drugs					
Erythromycin	Numerous	PO: 250, 333, 500 mg tab and cap IV	Diabetic gastroparesis	PO: 250–500 every 6 h IV: 500 mg every 6 h	
Metoclopramide	Reglan	IV PO: 10 mg tab	Diabetic gastroparesis Esophageal reflux	IV: 10 mg over 2 min PO: 10 mg 30 min before each meal and at bedtime	Restlessness Drowsiness Fatigue

HEMATOLOGIC DRUGS

GENERIC NAME	TRADE NAME	PREPARATIONS	GENERAL INDICATIONS	USUAL DOSAGE	CAUTIONS/COMMENTS
Antianemics Cyanocobalamin (Vitamin B$_{12}$)	Betalin-12 Redisol Others Generic	IM IV SC	Pernicious anemia	IM, IV, SC: 30–50 µg daily for 5–10 days, followed by 100 µg monthly	Patients with neurologic symptoms require higher doses on initiation of therapy
Ferrous fumarate	Feostat Ircon Toleron Generic	PO: 150, 200, 325 mg (33.3, 66, 107 mg elemental iron, respectively)	Iron deficiency anemia	PO: 1–4 tabs per day in divided doses (33 to 133 mg elemental iron/day)	GI symptoms can be reduced by taking drug with food or by reducing dose Nonprescription
Ferrous gluconate	Fergon Generic	PO: 435 mg cap (52 mg elemental iron) 320 mg tab (40 mg elemental iron)	Iron deficiency anemia	PO: 2–6 tabs per day in divided doses	GI symptoms can be reduced by taking drug with food
Ferrous sulfate	Feosol Fer-in-Sol Others Generic	PO: 150 mg cap (30 mg elemental iron) 192, 325 mg tab (39 and 65 mg of elemental iron, respectively) Numerous dosage strengths available	Iron deficiency anemia	PO: 1–4 tabs per day in divided doses (60–240 mg of elemental iron/day)	GI symptoms can be reduced by taking drug with food or by reducing dose Nonprescription
Folate sodium	Folvite solution	IV IM SC	Megaloblastic anemia	IV, IM, SC: up to 1 mg daily	May mask diagnosis of Vitamin B$_{12}$ deficiency

Table continued on following page

245

GENERIC NAME	TRADE NAME	PREPARATIONS	GENERAL INDICATIONS	USUAL DOSAGE	CAUTIONS/COMMENTS
Folic acid	Folvite Generic	PO: 0.1, 0.25, 0.4, 0.8, 1 mg tab	Megaloblastic anemia	PO: 0.25–1 mg daily	
Anticoagulants					
Dicumarol		PO: 25, 50, 100 mg cap 25, 50, 100 mg tab	Anticoagulation	PO: 75–100 mg daily for 3 days followed by 25–150 mg daily Adjust dosage with prothrombin time	Flatulence and diarrhea Maintain prothrombin activity at approximately 25% of normal or 2 times control
Heparin		IV Subcutaneous	Anticoagulation DIC	Must be individualized dosage given in units	Hemorrhage
Protamine sulfate		IV	Antidote for heparin excess	Each mg neutralizes approximately 80 units of heparin	Overdosage promotes hemorrhage Heparin package insert should be consulted
Warfarin	Coumadin Panwarfin Generic	IV IM PO: 2, 2.5, 5, 7.5, 10, 25 mg tab	Anticoagulation	IV, IM: Rarely used PO: 10–15 mg daily for 3 days followed by maintenance dose of 2–10 mg Adjust dosage with prothrombin time	Maintain prothrombin activity at approximately 1.2–2 times control Drug of choice for oral anticoagulation
Antiplatelet Drugs					
Aspirin	Generic	PO: 80, 325 mg tab	TIA Coronary artery disease	PO: 1 tablet daily	Optimal dose uncertain
Dipyridamole	Persantine	PO: 25, 50, 75 mg tab	TIA Coronary artery disease	PO: 75 mg–100 mg 3 times daily (or 100 mg/day with 1 aspirin)	Peripheral vasodilation Optimal dose uncertain

Sulfinpyrazone	Anturane	PO: 100, 200 mg tab	TIA Coronary artery disease	PO: 200 mg 3 to 4 times daily	GI disturbance
Ticlopidine	Ticlid	PO: 250 mg tab	TIA Secondary prevention of stroke	PO: 250 mg twice daily with food	GI disturbance Neutropenia Thrombocytopenia Rash

BLOOD COMPONENTS

Component	Usual Components	Comments
Albumin	20, 50, 100 ml 25% solution 250, 500 ml 5% solution	Contains no active clotting factors Useful as volume expander
Commercial concentrate of antihemophilic factor*	Vials contain 200–1000 Factor VIII units	Prepared from large pool of donors Risk of hepatitis is high
Commercial Factor IX*	Vial contains 500 Factor II, VII, IX, X units	Used in treatment of hemophilia B when plasma will not suffice or in hemophilia A patients who have developed inhibitors Risk of hepatitis is high
Cryoprecipitate*	100 Factor VIII units per bag containing 15–25 ml plasma	Bags are pooled and usual dose is 10–12 bags infused over 15–30 min
Leukopoor red blood cells*	Variable	Costly to prepare and should be used only in patients with febrile reactions to regular transfusion of whole blood or packed cells

*Risk of hepatitis is present.

Table continued on following page

Component	Usual Components	Comments
Packed red blood cells*	250 ml units with 200 ml cells and 50 ml plasma	Reduced risk of volume overload
Plasma*	200–250 ml units	Useful in bleeding disorders such as Factor IX deficiency Usually prepared as fresh frozen plasma to help facilitate storage
Platelets*	30–50 ml plasma with concentrated platelets	Units are pooled and should be kept at room temperature and used as soon as possible. Effectiveness should be assessed with a follow-up platelet count after 1, 4, and 24 hours. Usual dosage is 4–6 units, and a 10,000-count increment per unit is expected (in the absence of immunologic destruction or splenomegaly)

*Risk of hepatitis is present.

INFECTIOUS DISEASE DRUGS

GENERIC NAME	TRADE NAME	PREPARATIONS	GENERAL INDICATIONS	USUAL DOSAGE	CAUTIONS / COMMENTS
Antibacterial Agents					
Aminoglycosides					
Amikacin	Amikin	IV IM	Should be reserved for serious gram-negative infection resulting from strains known to be resistant to gentamicin or tobramycin	IV, IM: 7.5 mg/kg every 12 h	Side effects are similar for all aminoglycosides
Gentamicin	Garamycin	IV IM	Suspected gram-negative infections, including *Pseudomonas*	IV, IM: 1–1.7 mg/kg every 8 h	Side effects include ototoxicity, vestibular toxicity, nephrotoxicity Must reduce dosage if renal failure is present
Kanamycin	Kantrex	IV IM	Not active against *Pseudomonas*; therefore, gentamicin is preferred	IV, IM: 7.5 mg/kg every 12 h	Must reduce dosage if renal failure is present
Neomycin	Mycifradin Neobiotic	PO: 500 mg tab	Bowel sterilization, especially for hepatic precoma	PO: 1 g every 4–6 h	Absorption is minimal
Netilmicin	Netromycin	IV IM		IV, IM: 2–3 mg/kg every 12 h	Must reduce dosage if renal failure is present *Table continued on following page*

GENERIC NAME	TRADE NAME	PREPARATIONS	GENERAL INDICATIONS	USUAL DOSAGE	CAUTIONS / COMMENTS
Tobramycin	Nebcin	IV IM	Similar to gentamicin	IV, IM: 1–1.7 mg/kg every 8 h	Must reduce dosage if renal failure is present
Cephalosporins		Cephalosporins are generally used for serious infections from susceptible organisms. When the patient is sensitive to penicillin; cross sensitivity can occur, but it is uncommon			
FIRST GENERATION CEPHALOSPORINS					
Cefadroxil	Duricef Ultracef	PO: 500 mg cap		PO: 1 g every 12 h	First generation cephalosporins are not useful for meningitis
Cefazolin	Ancef Kefzol	IV IM		IV, IM: 500–1500 mg every 8 h	
Cephalexin	Keflex Ceporex	PO: 250, 500 mg cap		PO: 500 mg every 6 h	
Cephalothin	Keflin	IV		IV: 1 g every 4 h	
Cephapirin	Cefadyl	IV IM		IV, IM: 500 mg–1 g every 4–6 h	
Cephradine	Anspor Velosef	IV IM PO: 250, 500 mg cap		IV, IM: 500 mg–1 g every 4–6 hr PO: 250–500 mg	
SECOND GENERATION CEPHALOSPORINS					
Cefaclor	Ceclor	PO: 250, 500 mg cap		PO: 250 mg every 8 h	May be useful in treating ampicillin-resistant *H. influenzae*, otitis media, and respiratory infections

Generic	Trade	Route	Dosage	Comments
Cefamandole	Mandol	IV IM	IV, IM: 1-2 g every 6-8 h	Cefamandole, cefotetan, cefoxitin, and cefuroxime have increased activity against some gram-negative and anaerobic organisms as compared with other cephalosporins
Ceforanide	Precef	IV IM	IV, IM: 0.5-1.0 g every 12 h	
Cefotetan	Cefotan	IV IM	IV, IM: 1-2 g every 12 h	
Cefoxitin	Mefoxin	IV IM	IV, IM: 1-2 g every 6-8 h	
Cefuroxime	Zinacef	IV IM	IV, IM: 0.75 mg-1.5 g every 8 h	
THIRD GENERATION CEPHALOSPORINS				
Cefonicid	Monocid	IV IM	IV, IM: 1 g every day 2 g for severe infections	
Cefoperazone	Cefobid	IV IM	IV, IM: 1-2 g every 12 h	
Cefotaxime	Claforan	IV IM	IV, IM: 1-2 g every 6-8 h	
Ceftazidime	Tazidime Fortaz	IV IM	IV, IM: 1-2 g every 8 h	
Ceftizoxime	Cefizox	IV IM	IV,. IM: 1-2 g every 12 h	
Ceftriaxone	Rocephin	IV IM	IV, IM: 1-2 g every day	250 mg IM is effective for gonorrhea

Table continued on following page

GENERIC NAME	TRADE NAME	PREPARATIONS	GENERAL INDICATIONS	USUAL DOSAGE	CAUTIONS / COMMENTS
Moxalactam	Moxam	IV IM		IV, IM: 1–2 g every 8 h	
Cephalosporin-Related Drugs					
Aztreonam	Azactam	IV IM		IV: 1–2 g every 8–12 h	Active only against aerobic gram-negative bacilli No nephrotoxicity
Imipenem/cilastatin	Primaxin	IV	Serious infections	IV: 500 mg every 6 h	Active against β-lactamase production Seizures (especially with coexistent renal impairment)
Chloramphenicol Group					
Chloramphenicol	Chloromycetin Mychel Generic	IV PO: 50, 100, 250 mg cap	For ampicillin-resistant *H. influenzae*, bacteroides, typhoid fever	IV: PO: 500 mg every 6 h	Aplastic anemia, leukopenia (both idiosyncratic and dose-related)
Erythromycin Group					
Erythromycin	Many names and derivatives, all with the same activity	PO: 125, 250, 500 Estolate form often tolerated better with food	Useful alternative drug to penicillin for mild infections—not recommended for gonorrhea	PO: 250–500 mg every 6 h IV, IM: 500 mg every 6 h	Stearate form should be taken on empty stomach Enteric-coated base may be taken with food Erythromycin may cause cholestatic jaundice
Clindamycin	Cleocin	IV IM PO: 75, 150 mg cap	Serious anaerobic infections and treatment of some staphylococcal infections in patients who are allergic to penicillin	PO: 150–300 mg every 6 h IV: 200–400 mg every 8 h	Pseudomembranous enterocolitis is a rare side effect with clindamycin IM use is painful

Methenamines				
Methenamine	Generic	PO: 300, 500 mg tab	PO: 1 g 4 times daily	Methenamines are used for prophylaxis of chronic urinary tract infections
Methenamine mandelate	Mandelamine Generic	PO: 250, 500 mg 1 g tab	PO: 1 g 4 times daily	They require an acid urine (pH <5.5) for effectiveness
Methenamine hippurate	Hiprex Urex	PO: 1 g tab	PO: 1 g twice daily	Cranberry juice, prunes, plums, and ascorbic acid, 1 g 4 times daily, can be added to assure an acid urine
Methenamine sulfosalicylate	Hexalet	PO: 500 mg, 1 g tab	PO: 1 g 4 times daily	
Nalidixic Acid				
Nalidixic acid	NegGram	PO: 250, 500 mg tab	PO: 1 g 4 times daily	Urinary tract infection · Organisms often develop resistance to nalidixic acid after 24 h
Nitrofurans				
Nitrofurantoin	Furadantin Macrodantin Cyantin Generic	PO: 50, 100 mg tab Macrocrystalline form available in 25, 50, 100 mg cap	PO: 50–100 mg 4 times daily with food	Chronic or recurrent urinary tract infections · GI disturbances are less common with macrocrystalline forms · Dosage is lower when used for suppression
Penicillins				
Penicillin G	Many Generic	IV	IV: 250,000–2 million units every 2–6 h	
Procaine penicillin G	Many Generic	IM	IM: 600,000 units every 12 h	

Table continued on following page

GENERIC NAME	TRADE NAME	PREPARATIONS	GENERAL INDICATIONS	USUAL DOSAGE	CAUTIONS / COMMENTS
Benzathine penicillin G	Bicillin C-R Bicillin L-A Bicillin C-R 900/300 Permapen	IM		IM: 1.2 million units monthly for rheumatic heart disease prophylaxis	Permapen and Bicillin L-A contain only benzathine Bicillin C-R contains half benzathine and half procaine Bicillin C-R 900/300 contains 900,000 units of benzathine and 300,000 units of procaine in 2 ml
Penicillin V (phenoxymethyl penicillin)	Many Generic	PO: Many sizes, 250 mg = 400,000 units		PO: 250 mg every 6 h	Better absorption on empty stomach
Broad-Spectrum Penicillins					
Amdinocillin	Coactin	IV IM		IV: 10 mg/kg every 4 h	Indicated for serious UTI; not active against *Pseudomonas* or gram-positive bacteria
Amoxicillin	Amoxil Larotid Polymox Generic	PO: 250, 500 mg cap	Same as ampicillin, except that amoxicillin is not effective against shigella	PO: 250–500 mg every 8 h	Amoxicillin causes less diarrhea than PO ampicillin
Amoxicillin/Clavulanate	Augmentin	PO: 250, 500 mg tab		PO: 250 mg tab every 8 hr: 500 mg tab every 8 h for more serious infections	Active against β-lactamase production
Ampicillin	Many Generic	IV IM PO: Many sizes, 250, 500 mg cap	Meningitis and urinary tract, respiratory, GI, and otitis media infections	IV, IM: 500 mg–1 g every 6 h PO: 500 mg every 6 h	Haemophilus resistance increasingly common with ampicillin
Ampicillin/Sulbactam	Unasyn	IV IM		IV: 1.5–3 g every 6 h IM: 1.5–3 g every 6 h	Active against β-lactamase production

Azlocillin	Azlin	IV		IV: 2 g every 6 h; 4 g every 6 h for serious infections	Similar to carbenicillin Expanded *Pseudomonas* coverage
Carbenicillin	Geopen	IM PO: 382 mg tab	IV: Severe infection (anaerobes, *Pseudomonas*) IM, PO: Urinary tract infections	IV: 5 g every 4 h IM: 1–2 g every 6 h PO: 1–2 tabs 4 times daily	Serum levels with oral administration are too low for systemic infections Can cause sodium excess
Cloxacillin	Tegopen Cloxapen	PO: 250, 500 mg cap	Useful when staphylococcal infection is suspected	PO: 500 mg every 6 h	
Dicloxacillin	Dynapen Dycil	PO: 125, 250, 500 mg cap	Useful when staphylococcal infection is suspected	PO: 250–500 mg every 6 h	
Methicillin	Staphcillin Celbenin	IV	Useful when staphylococcal infection is suspected	IV: 1–2 g every 4 h	Interstitial nephritis
Mezlocillin	Mezlin	IV IM	IV: Severe infections IM: Urinary infections	IV: 3–4 g every 6 h for serious infections IM: 1.5–2 g every 6 h	Similar to carbenicillin
Nafcillin	Unipen	IV IM PO: 250, 500 mg cap	Useful when staphylococcal infection is suspected	IV, IM: 1–2 g every 4–6 h PO: 500 mg every 6 h	Interstitial nephritis Do not give oral form with meals IM route is painful
Oxacillin	Prostaphlin	IV IM PO: 250, 500 mg cap	Useful when staphylococcal infection is suspected	IV, IM: 1 g every 4 h PO: 500 mg every 6 h	Interstitial nephritis Do not give oral form with meals IM route is painful
Piperacillin	Pipracil	IV IM	IV: Severe infections IM: Urinary infections	IV: 3 g every 4–6 h IM: 2 g every 6 h	
Ticarcillin	Ticar	IV IM	Severe infection (anaerobes, *Pseudomonas*)	IV, IM: 75 mg every 6 h	
Ticarcillin/ Clavulanate	Timentin	IV		IV: 3 g every 4–6 h	Active against β-lactamase production

Table continued on following page

GENERIC NAME	TRADE NAME	PREPARATIONS	GENERAL INDICATIONS	USUAL DOSAGE	CAUTIONS / COMMENTS
Polymyxins					
Colistimethate	Coly-Mycin	IV IM	Polymyxins are used for serious urinary tract infections with organisms resistant to gentamicin or carbenicillin	IV, IM: 1 mg/kg every 8 h	IM route is painful
Polymyxin B	Aerosporin	IV IM		IV, IM: 1 mg/kg every 12 h	IM route is painful
Quinolones					
Ciprofloxacin	Cipro	PO: 250, 500, 750 mg tab IV	Severe infection with aerobic gram-negative rods Urinary tract infection with gram-negative bacilli resistant to other agents	PO: 500 mg b.i.d. IV: 400 mg every 12 h	Oral agent active against most *Pseudomonas aeruginosa* Adjust dosage in renal impairment
Norfloxacin	Noroxin	PO: 400 mg tab	Urinary tract infection with gram-negative bacilli resistant to other agents	PO: 400 mg b.i.d.	Reduced tissue bioavailability as compared to ciprofloxacin Use restricted to treatment of urinary tract infection
Ofloxacin	Floxin	PO: 200, 300, 400 mg tab	Similar to ciprofloxacin	PO: 200–400 mg b.i.d.	Similar to ciprofloxacin Also active against *Chlamydia trachomatis*
Spectinomycin					
Spectinomycin	Trobicin	IM	Gonorrhea in patient who fails to respond to penicillin, amoxicillin, cephtriaxone, ampicillin, or tetracycline	IM: 2 g in single dose	

Sulfonamides					
Sulfacetamide	Sulamyd	Ophthalmic ointment (10%) or solution (10%, 30%)	Bacterial conjunctivitis	1 drop applied 4 times daily	
Sulfamethizole	Thiosulfil	PO: 250, 500 mg tab	Urinary tract infections	PO: 1 g every 6 h	
Sulfamethoxazole	Gantanol	PO: 500 mg tab; double-strength tab available	Urinary tract infections	PO: 2 g loading dose, then 1 g every 12 h	Greater tendency to cause crystalluria than sulfisoxazole
Sulfisoxazole	Gantrisin Generic	IV PO: 500 mg tab	Urinary tract infections	IV: 25 mg/kg every 6 h PO: 2 g loading dose, then 1 g every 6 h	
Tetracyclines Tetracycline	Achromycin Panmycin Sumycin Others Generic	IV PO: 125, 250, 500 mg cap	For all tetracyclines: Suspected mycoplasmal pneumonia Rocky Mountain spotted fever Gonorrhea Nongonococcal urethritis	IV, PO: 250–500 mg every 6 h	Should be avoided in children and pregnant women unless specifically indicated
Chlortetracycline	Aureomycin	IV PO: 250 mg cap		IV, PO: 250–500 mg every 6 h	Should be avoided in children and pregnant women unless specifically indicated
Demeclocycline	Declomycin	IV PO: 75, 150, 300 mg tab; 150 mg cap		IV, PO: 150 mg every 6 h	Should be avoided in children and pregnant women unless specifically indicated
Doxycycline	Vibramycin	IV PO: 50, 100 mg cap		IV, PO: 100 mg every 12 h	Can be used in the presence of renal failure
Methacycline	Rondomycin	IV PO: 150, 300 mg cap		IV, PO: 150 mg every 6 h	Should be avoided in children and pregnant women unless specifically indicated

Table continued on following page

GENERIC NAME	TRADE NAME	PREPARATIONS	GENERAL INDICATIONS	USUAL DOSAGE	CAUTIONS / COMMENTS
Minocycline	Minocin Vectrin	IV PO: 50, 100 mg cap		IV, PO: 200 mg initially, then 100 mg every 12 h	Can be used in the presence of renal failure Vestibular dysfunction
Oxytetracycline	Terramycin	IV PO: 125, 250 mg cap		IV, PO: 250–500 mg every 6 h	Should be avoided in children and pregnant women unless specifically indicated
Trimethoprim Trimethoprim	Proloprim Trimpex	PO: 100 mg tab	Urinary tract infections	PO: 100 mg every 12 h	Rash, pruritus (3% incidence)
Trimethoprim and Sulfamethoxazole Trimethoprim and sulfamethoxazole	Septra Bactrim	IV PO: 80 mg trimethoprim, 400 mg sulfamethoxazole tab; double-strength tab available	Urinary tract infections Shigellosis *Pneumocystis carinii* pneumonia	PO: 2 tabs every 12 h or 1 double-strength tab every 12 h IV: 10–20 mg/kg daily given in 3–4 doses	
Vancomycin Vancomycin	Vancocin	IV PO: Powder for aqueous solution	Should be reserved for treatment of methicillin-resistant staphylococcal infections or enterococcal endocarditis in penicillin-allergic patients	IV: 1 g every 12 h PO: 125 mg every 6 h	Oral form useful for pseudomembranous colitis due to toxigenic *Clostridium difficile* IV use may cause thrombophlebitis
Antifungal Agents Amphotericin B	Fungizone	IV Intrathecal	Life-threatening systemic fungal infections	Complicated dosage schedule—consult PDR or package insert	

Drug	Trade Name	Indications	Preparations	Dosage	Comments
Clotrimazole	Lotrimin Gyne-Lotrimin	Intradermal dermatophytes *Candida*	Topical: Cream 1% and solution 1% Vaginal: 100 mg tab	Topical: Apply to affected area twice daily Vaginal: One tablet inserted nightly for 1 week	Vaginal tablets come with applicator
Fluconazole	Diflucan	Mucocutaneous and systemic candidiasis *Coccidioides immitis* Cryptococcal infections	PO: 50, 100, 200 mg tab IV	PO/IV: 100–400 mg/day	Adjust dosage in renal failure GI absorption not affected by elevated gastric pH
Flucytosine	Ancobon	Used in combination with amphotericin B for selected systemic fungal infections	PO: 250, 500 mg cap	PO: 35 mg/kg every 6 h	Use with caution in patients in renal failure
Griseofulvin	Fulvicin-U/F Grisactin Others Generic	Intradermal dermatophytes, onychomycosis	PO: (Microcrystalline) 125, 250, 500 mg tab PO: (Ultramicrocrystalline) 125 mg tab	PO: (Micro) 500 mg– 1 g/day single dose PO: (Ultramicro) 250–500 mg/day single dose	Not active against *Candida*
Ketoconazole	Nizoral	Chronic mucocutaneous candidiasis	PO: 200 mg tab	PO: 200–400 mg daily	GI disturbances Elevated gastric pH decreases absorption
Miconazole	Micatin Monistat i.v.	Intradermal dermatophytes *Candida* IV route used for selected serious systemic infections	IV Topical: 2% cream Vaginal: 2% cream with applicator	Topical: Apply to affected area twice daily Vaginal: One applicatorful nightly for 2 weeks IV: Dosage varies with organism—consult PDR or package insert	Topical is OTC

Table continued on following page

GENERIC NAME	TRADE NAME	PREPARATIONS	GENERAL INDICATIONS	USUAL DOSAGE	CAUTIONS / COMMENTS
Nystatin	Mycostatin Nilstat	PO: 500,000 units tab or suspension Topical: Cream and ointment 100,000 units/g in 15 g containers	*Candida* infections of skin, mucous membranes, GI tract, and vagina	PO: 1–2 tabs 3 times daily or 4–6 ml suspension, swish in mouth Topical: Apply to affected area twice daily Vaginal: 1–2 tabs daily for 2 weeks	
Tolnaftate	Tinactin	Topical: 1% solution, cream, powder, and aerosol	Intradermal dermatophytes	Topical: Apply to affected area twice daily	Nonprescription
Antiparasitic Agents					
Crotamiton	Eurax	Topical: 10% cream in 60 g containers	Scabies	Topical: Massage into skin from chin to feet; repeat in 24 h	
Furazolidone	Furoxone	PO: 100 mg tab	Giardiasis	PO: 100 mg q.i.d. for 7–10 days	Occasional GI side effects
Gamma benzene	Kwell Gamene	Topical: 1% cream, lotion, shampoo	Scabies Pediculosis	Topical: Apply to entire body (except face); wash off after 24 h Shampoo: Lather 1 oz into scalp, allow to remain 5 min, then rinse thoroughly	May repeat application in 4 days
Iodoquinol	Diquinol Yodoquinol Yodoxin	PO: 210, 650 mg tab	Amebiasis	PO: 650 mg PO t.i.d. for 20 days	Active against both the cysts and trophozoites of *Entamoeba histolytica*

Mebendazole	Vermox	PO: 100 mg tab	Roundworm Whipworm Hookworm Pinworm	PO: 100 mg every 12 h for 3 days For pinworms: 100 mg in single dose	A second course may be required in 3 weeks
Metronidazole	Flagyl Metryl	IV PO: 250, 500 mg tab	Amebiasis Giardiasis Trichomonas	PO: For amebiasis and giardiasis: 750 mg 3 times daily for 5–10 days For trichomonas: Single 2 g dose or 250 mg 3 times daily for 7 days	Avoid in pregnant women Do not take with alcohol
Paromomycin	Humatin	PO: 250 mg cap	Amebiasis, and possibly other intestinal protozoa Cestodes	PO: For amebiasis: 25–35 mg/kg daily in 3 divided doses For cestodes: 1 gram every 15 minutes for 14 doses	A nonabsorbable aminoglycoside
Pentamidine	Pentam	IV	*Pneumocystis carinii* pneumonia African trypanosomiasis Visceral leishmaniasis	IV: For *Pneumocystis carinii*: 3–4 mg/kg qd for 14–21 days	Possible side effects include nephrotoxicity, hypoclycemia, hypotension, and neutropenia Inhaled preparation available for *Pneumocystis carinii* prophylaxis
Praziquantel	Biltricide	PO: 600 mg tab	Schistosomiasis and other infections with trematodes Cestodes (including neurocysticercosis)	PO: For schistosomiasis: 60 mg/kg every 6 h for 3 doses For neurocysticercosis: 50 mg/kg in 3 divided doses for 14–21 days	Treatment of neurocysticercosis should be initiated in the hospital; adverse CNS effects (e.g., seizures, headache) reduced by administration of corticosteroids

Table continued on following page

GENERIC NAME	TRADE NAME	PREPARATIONS	GENERAL INDICATIONS	USUAL DOSAGE	CAUTIONS / COMMENTS
Pyrantel pamoate	Antiminth	PO: 250 mg/5 ml liquid	Pinworms Roundworms Hookworms	PO: For pinworms and roundworms: 11 mg/kg single dose (up to 1 g) For hookworms: 11 mg/kg daily for 3 days (up to 1 g)	
Quinacrine	Atabrine	PO: 100 mg tab	Giardiasis	PO: 100 mg 3 times daily for 5 days	Preferred over metronidazole for pregnant women
Thiabendazole	Mintezol	PO: 500 mg tab	Cutaneous larva migrans Strongyloidiasis	PO: 3 tab 2 times a day for 2 days	Adjust for weight of patient
Antituberculosis Agents					
Ethambutol	Myambutol	PO: 100, 400 mg tab	Used in combination therapy	PO: 15 mg/kg/day in single dose	Optic neuritis generally occurs at dosages above 15 mg/kg/day
Isoniazid	INH Hyzyd Niconyl Others	PO: 100, 300 mg tab	Used in combination therapy or alone for prophylaxis	PO: 300 mg/day in single dose	Incidence of hepatitis is age-related Can cause peripheral neuropathy related to pyridoxine deficiency
Pyrazinamide		PO: 500 mg tab	Used in combination therapy	PO: 15–30 mg/kg (up to 2 g) daily	Possible hepatotoxicity
Rifampin	Rifadin Rimactane	PO: 300 mg cap	Used in combination therapy	PO: 600 mg/day in single dose	Elevated SGOT and bilirubin (usually transient)
Streptomycin		IM	Tuberculosis	IM: 15–25 mg/kg/day in 2 divided doses	

Antiviral Agents

Acyclovir	Zovirax	PO: 200 mg cap IV Topical	Primary herpes simplex Recurrent herpes simplex Disseminated varicella-zoster	PO: 200 mg every 4 h (5 cap daily) for 10 days (for primary herpes) IV: 5 mg/kg given over 1 h 3 times daily (for herpes simplex) For herpes encephalitis: 12.5–15 mg/kg 3 times daily	Should be used only in proven infection
Adenine arabinoside	Vira-A	IV Ophthalmic: 3% ointment	Herpes simplex encephalitis and keratoconjunctivitis	IV: 15 mg/kg/day diluted in 500–1000 ml D5W given slowly over 12 h for 10 days	
Amantadine	Symmetrel	PO: 100 mg cap	For prophylaxis and treatment of influenza A	PO: 100 mg daily	May be of benefit in early influenza A infection Not of benefit for influenza B
Didanosine	Videx	PO: 25, 50, 100, 150 mg tab	For treatment of HIV infection in patients intolerant of zidovudine	PO: 100–200 mg/kg b.i.d.	Adjust dosage according to weight Toxicity includes pancreatitis, peripheral neuropathy, and GI side effects Minimal myelosuppression
Ganciclovir	Cytovene	IV	Cytomegalovirus infections	IV: Induction: 5 mg/kg every 12 h Maintenance: 5–6 mg/kg daily for 5–7 days/week	Bone marrow suppression Adjust dosage in renal failure
Zidovudine	Retrovir	PO: 100 mg cap IV	HIV infection (AIDS or CD4 count less than 500/mm³)	PO: 100 mg PO5 times daily or 100–200 mg t.i.d.	Toxicity includes bone marrow suppression, GI side effects, headache, malaise, and myalgia/myositis

NEUROLOGIC DRUGS

GENERIC NAME	TRADE NAME	PREPARATIONS	GENERAL INDICATIONS	USUAL DOSAGE	CAUTIONS/COMMENTS
Agents for Migraine					
Ergotamine tartrate	Ergomar Gynergen	IM SC PO: 1 mg tab 2 mg sublingual tab Medihaler form available containing 0.36 mg per inhalation	Acute attack of migraine Most effective when given soon after onset Also helpful for cluster headache when 1–2 mg taken at bedtime for 10–14 days	IM, SC: 0.25–0.5 mg at onset of attack, may repeat in 40 min (up to 1 mg in one week) PO: 1–2 mg at onset, then 1–2 mg every 30 min (up to 6 mg in 24 h and 10 mg in one week) Sublingual: 2 mg at onset and 1–2 mg every 30 min (up to 6 mg in 24 h and 10 mg in one week)	Contraindicated in patients with peripheral vascular disease
Methysergide maleate	Sansert	PO: 2 mg tab	Prophylaxis of migraine and cluster headaches	PO: 4–6 mg daily in individual doses, taken with food	Of no value in acute attacks Serious adverse reactions include retroperitoneal fibrosis

264

Propranolol	Inderal	PO: 10, 20, 40, 80 mg tab	Prophylaxis of migraine	PO: 80 mg daily in divided doses Usual effective range: 160–240 mg daily	Stop after 4–6 weeks if there has been no satisfactory response Discontinue therapy gradually over 2–3 weeks Contraindicated in patients with CHF and asthma
Sumatriptan	Imitrex	SC: 6 mg	Acute attack of migraine	SC: Self administered 6 mg injection; repeated dose not more effective; lower dose may work	Tingling Dizziness Flushing Warm/hot sensations
Combinations for Migraine Ergotamine, caffeine	Cafergot Generic	PO: Tab (1 mg ergotamine and 100 mg caffeine) Suppository: 2 mg ergotamine and 100 mg caffeine	Acute attack of migraine	PO: 2 tabs at onset of attack, then one tab every 30 min (up to 6 tabs in 24 h and 10 tabs in 1 week) Suppository: 1 at onset, may repeat in 1 h up to 2 suppositories per attack and 5 in 1 week	See *ergotamine*
Ergotamine, caffeine, pentobarbital, belladonna	Cafergot P-B	PO: Tab (same as Cafergot plus 30 mg pentobarbital and 0.125 mg belladonna) Suppository: Same as Cafergot plus 60 mg pentobarbital	Acute attack of migraine	PO: Same as Cafergot Suppository: Same as Cafergot	

Table continued on following page

GENERIC NAME	TRADE NAME	PREPARATIONS	GENERAL INDICATIONS	USUAL DOSAGE	CAUTIONS/COMMENTS
Agents for Vertigo					
Meclizine	Antivert Bonine	PO: 12.5, 25 mg tab	Vertigo of vestibular origin Motion sickness	For motion sickness: 25–50 mg 1 h before travel For vertigo: 25–100 mg daily	Drowsiness
Anticonvulsants					
Carbamazepine	Tegretol	PO: 200 mg tab	Generalized tonic clonic seizures Simple and complex partial seizures	PO: 200 mg twice daily initially, with 200 mg increment as needed Usual maintenance	Bone marrow suppression Sedation
Clonazepam	Clonopin	PO: 0.5, 1, 2 mg tab	Absence seizures Myoclonic and akinetic seizures resistant to other agents	PO: 1.5 mg daily in 3 divided doses; may increase by 0.5 to 1.0 mg every 3 days (maximum 20 mg/day)	Drowsiness Ataxia Personality changes
Diazepam	Valium	IV IM PO: 2, 5, 10 mg tab	Status epilepticus Anxiety	IV: 5–10 mg (slowly)	Respiratory depression at high dosages
Ethosuximide	Zarontin	PO: 250 mg cap	Absence seizures	PO: 500 mg once daily	GI symptoms Eosinophilia in 10% of patients
Phenobarbital	Eskabarb Luminal Generic	IV IM PO: 7.5, 15, 30, 60, 100 mg tab	Generalized tonic clonic seizures Status epilepticus	For status epilepticus: IV, IM: 200–390 mg (slowly) For seizure prophylaxis: PO: 60 mg 3 times daily	Sedation Respiratory depression at high dosages

Phenytoin	Dilantin	IV IM PO: 30, 100 mg tab	Generalized tonic clonic seizures Arrhythmias (see under *Cardiovascular Drugs*)	For rapid dilantinization: IV: 50 mg/min up to 1 g PO: 500 mg every 12 h for one day Maintenance dose: 300 mg once daily	Hypotension and arrhythmias may occur at rapid IV dosage
Primidone	Mysoline	PO: 50, 250 mg tab	Substitute for phenobarbital for patients not responding to phenobarbital or phenytoin	PO: 250 mg (in single dose at bedtime) to 2 g daily (in divided doses)	Drowsiness Patients not previously treated with phenobarbital should be started at low doses (50–125 mg at bedtime)
Valproic acid	Depakene	PO: 250 mg cap	Absence seizures Generalized tonic clonic seizures	PO: 1–2 g per day (start at 250 mg b.i.d. and increase dose gradually every 3–7 days)	GI symptoms (usually transient)
Antiparkinsonism Agents					
Amantadine	Symmetrel	PO: 100 mg cap	Parkinsonism	PO: 100 mg initially after breakfast for 5 days; if tolerated, an additional 100 mg is given after lunch	Dizziness Nervousness Ataxia Livedo reticularis (especially in women)
Benztropine mesylate	Cogentin	IV IM PO: 0.5, 1, 2 mg tab	Drug-induced extrapyramidal reactions Parkinsonism	IV, IM: 2 mg PO: 0.5–1 mg initially, at bedtime; gradually increase to 4–6 mg daily, if required	IV use is preferred for acute extrapyramidal reactions

Table continued on following page

GENERIC NAME	TRADE NAME	PREPARATIONS	GENERAL INDICATIONS	USUAL DOSAGE	CAUTIONS/COMMENTS
Bromocriptine	Parlodel	PO: 2.5, 5 mg	Parkinsonism, not responding to Sinemet or levodopa	PO: 1.25 mg twice daily initially, increase gradually	Hypotension Nausea Headache Confusion Close physician supervision is required
Levodopa	Dopar Larodopa Generic	PO: 125, 250, 500 mg cap and tab	Parkinsonism	PO: Dosage must be individualized Usual initial daily dose: 300 mg–1 g given in divided doses with food Gradually increase dosage; optimal dosage is 4–6 g daily	
Levodopa and carbidopa	Sinemet	PO: Sinemet 10/100 (10 mg carbidopa and 100 mg levodopa) Sinemet 25/250 (25 mg carbidopa and 250 mg levodopa) Sinemet 25/100 also available	Parkinsonism	PO: Dosage must be individualized Initial daily dose: 3–4 tabs of Sinemet 10/100 Usual daily dose: 3–6 tabs of Sinemet 25/250	Close physician supervision is required
Selegiline	Eldepryl	PO: 5 mg tab	Adjunct to levodopa/carbidopa for parkinsonism	PO: 5 mg twice daily, breakfast and lunch	Should try to reduce dose of levodopa/carbidopa after 2–3 days treatment; nausea, dizziness, agitation, insomnia
Trihexyphenidyl	Artane Tremin	PO: 2, 5 mg tab, 5 mg cap	Drug-induced extrapyramidal reactions Parkinsonism	PO: 2 mg initially Gradually increase up to 20 mg, if required	Glaucoma Atropine-like side effects

PSYCHIATRIC DRUGS

GENERIC NAME	TRADE NAME	PREPARATIONS	GENERAL INDICATIONS	USUAL DOSAGE	CAUTIONS / COMMENTS
Antianxiety Agents: Most antianxiety drugs have abuse potential and may cause oversedation.					
Alprazolam	Xanax	PO: 0.25, 0.5, 1 mg	Anxiety	PO: 0.25–0.5 mg 3 times daily	Reduce dosage in elderly patients
Buspirone	BuSpar	PO: 5, 10 mg tab	Anxiety	PO: 5–10 mg b.i.d.–t.i.d.	Little if any potential for tolerance or physiologic dependence
Chlordiazepoxide	Librium Libritabs Generic	IV IM PO: 5, 10, 25 mg tab (Libritabs) 5, 10, 25 mg cap	Anxiety Alcohol withdrawal	For anxiety: PO: 5–25 mg twice daily or once daily at bedtime	Reduce dosage in elderly patients Oral administration is preferred
Clorazepate	Tranxene	PO: Tranxene: 3.75, 7.5, 15 mg cap 11.25, 22.5 mg tab Azene: 3.25, 6.5, 13 mg cap	Anxiety Alcohol withdrawal	PO: 15–60 mg (or 13–52 mg) daily divided into 2–4 doses or in single dose at bedtime	Reduce dosage in elderly patients
Diazepam	Valium	IV IM PO: 2, 5, 10 mg	Anxiety Seizures Alcohol withdrawal Muscle relaxant	IV, IM: 2–5 mg initially PO: 2–10 mg 1–4 times daily	Reduce dosage in elderly patients
Halazepam	Paxipam	PO: 20, 40 mg tab	Anxiety	PO: 20–40 mg 3 to 4 times daily	Reduce dosage in elderly patients *Table continued on following page*

GENERIC NAME	TRADE NAME	PREPARATIONS	GENERAL INDICATIONS	USUAL DOSAGE	CAUTIONS / COMMENTS
Hydroxyzine	Atarax Vistaril Generic	IM PO: 25, 50, 100 mg cap and tab	Anxiety Allergic dermatoses	For anxiety: IM: 50–100 mg every 4–6 h PO: 25–100 mg 3–4 times daily For allergic dermatoses: 25 mg PO 3–4 times daily	
Lorazepam	Ativan	PO: 0.5, 1, 2, mg tab	Anxiety	PO: 1–2 mg 2–3 times daily	Reduce dosage in elderly patients
Oxazepam	Serax	PO: 10, 15, 30 mg cap 15 mg tab	Anxiety	PO: 10–30 mg 3–4 times daily	Reduce dosage in elderly patients
Prazepam	Centrax Verstran	PO: 5, 10, mg cap (Centrax) 10 mg tab (Verstran)	Anxiety	PO: 20 mg daily in single dose	Reduce dosage in elderly patients
Antidepressants *Tricyclics*		The initial daily dose may be 50% to 100% higher for hospitalized patients. Dosages are usually increased gradually over 2 weeks until maximal effects are achieved.			
Amitriptyline	Elavil Endep Amitid SK- Amitriptyline	IM PO: 10, 25, 50, 75, 100, 150 mg tab	Depression	IM: 80–120 mg daily in divided doses PO: Maintenance dose: 50–150 mg daily at bedtime	Dosage must be individualized 1–4 weeks may elapse before improvement is noted High sedative effects as compared with other tricyclics
Amoxapine	Asendin	PO: 25, 50, 100, 150 mg tab	Depression	PO: Usual maintenance dose 50–200 mg daily	Dosage must be individualized

Drug	Brand Names	Dosage Forms	Indication	Dosage	Comments
Desipramine	Norpramin Pertofrane	PO: 10, 25, 50, 75, 100, 150 mg tab and cap	Depression	PO: Usual maintenance dose: 50–150 mg at bedtime	Dosage must be individualized 1–4 weeks may elapse before improvement is noted
Doxepin	Sinequan Adapin	PO: 10, 25, 50, 75, 100, 150 mg cap	Depression	PO: Usual maintenance dose: 50–150 mg at bedtime	Dosage must be individualized 1–4 weeks may elapse before improvement is noted High sedative effects as compared with other tricyclics
Imipramine	Tofranil-PM Tofranil Imavate SK-Pramine	IM PO: 10, 25, 50 mg tab 75, 100, 125, 150 mg cap (Tofranil-PM)	Depression	IM: Up to 100 mg daily in divided doses PO: Maintenance dose: 50–150 mg daily at bedtime	Dosage must be individualized 1–4 weeks may elapse before improvement is noted
Nortriptyline	Aventyl Pamelor	PO: 10, 25 mg cap	Depression	PO: Maintenance dose: 50–100 mg at bedtime	Dosage must be individualized 1–4 weeks may elapse before improvement is noted
Protriptyline	Vivactil Triptil	PO: 5, 10 mg tab	Depression	PO: Maintenance dose: 10–30 mg at bedtime	Dosage must be individualized 1–4 weeks may elapse before improvement is noted Little or no sedative effects
Trazodone	Desyrel	PO: 50, 100, 150, 300 mg tab	Depression	PO: 75–150 mg daily in divided doses up to 300 mg per day	Dosage must be individualized
Trimipramine	Surmontil	PO: 25, 50 mg tab	Depression	PO: 25 mg 3 times daily Maintenance dose: 50–150 mg at bedtime	Dosage must be individualized 1–4 weeks may elapse before improvement is noted High sedative effects as compared with other tricyclics

Table continued on following page

GENERIC NAME	TRADE NAME	PREPARATIONS	GENERAL INDICATIONS	USUAL DOSAGE	CAUTIONS / COMMENTS
Tetracyclic Maprotiline	Ludiomil	PO: 25, 50 mg tab	Depression	PO: Initially, 100–150 mg in divided doses	Dosage must be individualized
MAO Inhibitors Isocarboxazid	Marplan	PO: 10 mg tab	Depression	PO: 10 mg 3 times daily Maintenance dose: 10–20 mg daily	With MAO inhibitors, life-threatening severe hypertension may be precipitated by tyramine-containing foods (wine, beer, coffee, cheese, and yogurt) and sympathomimetic agents (found in many proprietary cold, hay fever, or weight-reducing preparations)
Phenelzine	Nardil	PO: 15 mg tab	Depression	PO: 45–75 mg daily in 3 divided doses	
Tranylcypromine	Parnate	PO: 10 mg tab	Depression	PO: 10 mg twice daily	
Combinations Containing Antidepressants with an Antipsychotic or Antianxiety Drug Chlordiazepoxide, amitriptyline	Limbitrol	PO: 5–12.5, 10–25 tabs 5–12.5 tabs contain 5 mg chlordiazepoxide and 12.5 mg amitriptyline 10–25 tabs contain 10 mg chlordiazepoxide and 25 mg amitriptyline	Psychoneurosis with anxiety and depression	PO: Dosage must be individualized Usual maintenance dose: 5–12.5 or 10–25 combination tabs 3–4 times daily	

Perphenazine, amitriptyline	Etrafon Triavil	PO: 2-10, 2-15 tabs 2-10 tabs contain 2 mg perphenazine and 10 mg amitriptyline 2-25 tabs contain 2 mg perphenazine 25 mg amitriptyline Also 4-10 and 4-25 combinations	Schizoaffective disorder with depression	PO: Dosage must be individualized Usual maintenance dose: 2-10 or 4-25 combination tabs 2–4 times daily	
Other Antidepressant Fluoxetene	Prozac	PO: 20 mg cap	Major depression	PO: 20–40 mg/day	Less sedating than other antidepressants
Antimanics Lithium carbonate	Eskalith Lithane Lithonate	PO: 300 mg cap and tab	Manic-depressive illness Depression	For acute mania: PO: 1.2–1.8 g daily in 3 divided doses Usual maintenance dose: 300 mg t.i.d.	Dosage must be individualized Serum level must not exceed 2 mEq/L Prior to initiation of therapy, patients should have a baseline evaluation of cardiovascular, renal, thyroid, electrolyte, and neurologic status Careful monitoring is required for patients receiving this drug Lithium should be avoided during pregnancy

Table continued on following page

GENERIC NAME	TRADE NAME	PREPARATIONS	GENERAL INDICATIONS	USUAL DOSAGE	CAUTIONS / COMMENTS
Antipsychotics	The development of tardive dyskinesia is a risk following the use of all traditional antipsychotic drugs. Extrapyramidal reactions, sedation, and autonomic side effects can also commonly occur. The dosages of these agents must be carefully individualized.				
Acetophenazine	Tindal	PO: 20 mg tab	Psychosis	PO: 60 mg initially daily in divided doses; increase every several days by 20 mg Usual maintenance dose: 80–120 mg daily	Use one-half the dosage for elderly patients
Butaperazine	Repoise	PO: 10, 25 mg tab	Psychosis	PO: 15–30 mg daily in 3 divided doses; increase weekly by 5–10 mg (maximum of 100 mg daily)	Use one-half the dosage for elderly patients
Chlorpromazine	Thorazine Others	IM PO: 10, 25, 50, 100, 220 mg tab Suppository: 25, 100 mg	Psychosis	PO: 200–600 mg initially daily in divided doses; increase every several days by 100 mg (up to 2 g/day)	Postural hypotension Use one-half the dosage for elderly patients IM use should be avoided, as other agents less likely to cause hypotension are available
Chlorprothixene	Taractan	IM PO: 10, 25, 50, 100 mg	Psychosis	IM: 75–200 mg daily in divided doses PO: 75–200 mg initially daily in divided doses; increase gradually up to maximum of 600 mg	Use one-half the dosage for elderly patients

Generic	Trade name	Preparation	Indications	Dosage	Comments
Fluphenazine decanoate Fluphenazine enanthate	Prolixin Decanoate Prolixin Enanthate	IM Depot preparation	Psychosis Useful for patients with poor cooperation or inadequate absorption of oral medications	IM: Usual maintenance dose: 12.5–100 mg every 2 weeks	Use one-half the dosage for elderly patients Extrapyramidal reactions may be difficult to control
Fluphenazine HCl	Prolixin Permitil	IM PO: 0.25, 1, 2.5, 5, 10 mg tab	Psychosis	For acute psychosis: IM: 1.25 mg initially; gradually increase to 2.5–10 mg daily in divided doses Usual maintenance dose: 1–5 mg daily PO: 2.5–10 mg initially Usual maintenance dose: 1–5 mg daily	Dosage must be individualized Use one-half the dosage for elderly patients 2 mg are equivalent to 100 mg chlorpromazine
Haloperidol	Haldol	IM PO: 0.5, 1, 2, 5, 10 mg tab	Psychosis and severe agitation Hyperkinetic states	For acute psychosis: IM: 2–5 mg every h For severe agitation: IM: 5–10 mg every h until controlled PO: 1–15 mg daily initially in divided doses Usual maintenance dose: 2–10 mg daily	Use one-half the dosage for elderly patients
Loxapine	Loxitane	PO: 5, 10, 25, 50 mg cap	Psychosis	PO: 10 mg twice daily; increase as needed Usual maintenance dose: 60–100 mg daily	Use one-half the dosage for elderly patients

Table continued on following page

GENERIC NAME	TRADE NAME	PREPARATIONS	GENERAL INDICATIONS	USUAL DOSAGE	CAUTIONS / COMMENTS
Mesoridazine	Serentil	IM PO: 10, 25, 50, 100 mg tab	Psychosis	PO: 150 mg initially daily in divided doses; increase every several days by 50 mg Usual maintenance dose: 100–400 mg daily	Use one-half the dosage for elderly patients IM route painful
Molindone	Lidone Moban	PO: 5, 10, 25 mg cap and tab	Psychosis	PO: 5–15 mg 3–4 times daily; gradually increase as needed	Use one-half the dosage for elderly patients
Perphenazine	Trilafon	IM PO: 2, 4, 8, 16 mg tab	Psychosis	For acute psychosis: IM: 5–10 mg initially then 5 mg every 6 h PO: 16–64 mg daily initially in divided doses	Use one-half the dosage for elderly patients
Piperacetazine	Quide	PO: 10, 25 mg tab	Psychosis	PO: 20–40 mg daily initially in divided doses	Use one-half the dosage for elderly patients
Thioridazine	Mellaril	PO: 10, 15, 25, 50, 100, 150, 200 mg tab	Psychosis	PO: 150–300 mg initially daily in divided doses; increase gradually up to 800 mg daily	Use one-half the dosage for elderly patients
Thiothixene	Navane	IM PO: 1, 2, 5, 10, 20 mg cap	Psychosis	For acute psychosis: IM: 4 mg 2–4 times daily; increase gradually up to 30 mg daily	Use one-half the dosage for elderly patients

Generic	Brand	Supplied	Indications	Dosage	Special Considerations
Trifluoperazine	Stelazine	IM PO: 1, 2, 5, 10 mg tab	Psychosis	PO: 6–10 mg daily initially in divided doses Usual maintenance dose: 20–30 mg daily For severe agitation: 10–20 mg PO every hour until controlled For acute psychosis: IM: 2–5 mg initially followed by 1–2 mg every 4–6 h PO: 2–4 mg initially daily in divided doses	Use one-half the dosage for elderly patients
Triflupromazine	Vesprin	IM PO: 10, 25, 50 mg	Psychosis	For acute psychosis: IM: 60–150 mg daily PO: 50–150 mg daily initially in divided doses	Use one-half the dosage for elderly patients

Non-Traditional Antipsychotic

Generic	Brand	Supplied	Indications	Dosage	Special Considerations
Clozapine	Clozaril	PO: 25, 100 mg tab	Severely ill schizophrenia unresponsive to traditional antipsychotics	Initiate 12.5–25 mg qd or bid, increase 25–50 mg/d to achieve target dose of 300–450 mg/d by 2 weeks; subsequent dose adjustments no more than once or twice weekly	*Life-threatening Granulocytopenia* Requires weekly WBC testing as condition of distribution; sedation, seizures tachycardia, hypotension

ANTIPSYCHOTIC DRUGS: SIDE EFFECTS AND RELATIVE POTENCY*

		Sedation	Autonomic	Extrapyramidal Reaction	Equivalent Oral Dose (mg)
Chlorpromazine	Thorazine	3+	2+	2+	100
Thioridazine	Mellaril	3+	3+	1+	100
Chlorprothixene	Taractan	3+	2+	1½+	100
Mesoridazine	Serentil	3+	2+	1+	50
Triflupromazine	Vesprin	3+	2½+	2+	25
Carphenazine	Proketazine	2+	1+	3+	25
Acetophenazine	Tindal	2+	1+	3+	20
Piperacetazine	Quide	2+	1+	2+	10
Molindone	Lidone, Moban	2+	2+	2½+	10
Loxapine	Daxolin, Loxitane	2+	1½+	3+	10
Butaperazine	Repoise	2+	1+	3+	10
Perphenazine	Trilafon	1½+	1+	3+	8
Trifluoperazine	Stelazine	2+	1+	3+	5
Thiothixene	Navane	1+	1+	3+	4
Haloperidol	Haldol	1+	1+	3+	2
Fluphenazine	Permitil, Prolixin	1½+	1+	3+	2

*Modified from AMA Drug Evaluation, 4th edition. Chicago, AMA, 1980.

RENAL DRUGS

GENERIC NAME	TRADE NAME	PREPARATIONS	GENERAL INDICATIONS	USUAL DOSAGE	CAUTIONS / COMMENTS
Agents to Correct Electrolyte and Mineral Abnormalities					
Calcitonin	Calcimar	IM SC	Hypercalcemia Emergencies Paget's disease	IM: 100–400 MRC units	Plicamycin is preferred for emergencies Skin test before using
Calcium carbonate	Tums, others	PO: Powder	Hypocalcemia	PO: 1–2 g 3 times daily	
Calcium chloride		IV: 10% solution	Severe hypocalcemia	IV: 5–10 ml of 10% solution	Avoid extravasation
Calcium gluceptate		IM IV	Severe hypocalcemia	IM: 2–5 ml in gluteal region IV: 10 ml	
Calcium gluconate		IV PO: 300, 600 mg tab	Hypocalcemia Severe hypocalcemia	IV: 20 ml of 10% solution injected slowly, followed by slow infusion PO: 15 g daily in divided doses	
Dihydrotachysterol (Vitamin D)	Hytakerol	PO: 0.2 mg tab 0.125 mg cap	Hypoparathyroidism	PO: 0.75–2.5 mg daily initially Maintenance dose: 0.25–1.75 mg weekly	Hypercalcemia may occur

Table continued on following page

279

GENERIC NAME	TRADE NAME	PREPARATIONS	GENERAL INDICATIONS	USUAL DOSAGE	CAUTIONS/ COMMENTS
Etidronate	Didronel	PO: 200, 400 mg tab IV	Paget's disease Heterotopic ossification Osteoporosis Hypercalcemia of malignant disease	PO: Paget's disease: 5–10 mg/kg/day for no longer than 6 months IV: Hypercalcemia of malignant disease: 7.5 mg/kg/day for 3–7 days	Relatively limited oral bioavailability Increased risk of fractures and osteomalacia with prolonged treatment
Magnesium sulfate		IM, IV: 10%, 25%, 50% solution	Hypomagnesemia	IM, IV: 2–4 g (16–32 mEq) in divided doses	
Plicamycin	Mithracin	IV	Hypercalcemia emergencies	IV: 25 µg/kg in D5W infused over 4–8 h	
Potassium chloride	K-Lor Slow-K Kay Ciel Elixir K-Lyte/CL Others	IV PO: Most liquid preparations contain 10–40 mEq per 15 ml	Hypokalemia	IV: Never inject undiluted Generally, rate should not exceed 10–15 mEq/h PO: 15–30 mEq daily Do not exceed 100–300 mEq/day	In extreme situations, faster infusion of IV solutions is permissible
Prednisone	See under *Endocrine Drugs*	PO: 10, 20, 40, 50 mg tab	Hypercalcemia	PO: 15 mg 4 times daily	Other corticosteroids are effective

Sodium polystyrene sulfonate	Kayexalate	Hyperkalemia	PO: Powder Rectal	PO: 15 g (in 200 ml water) 1–4 times daily Rectal: Retention enema, 30–80 g suspended in 150 ml to 200 ml D10W 1–3 times a day initially	Action is slow; therefore, other measures should be used in urgent circumstances
Phosphate Binders					
Aluminum carbonate	Basaljel	Antacid Phosphate binder	PO: Suspension, capsules, tablets	PO: 2 caps or tabs 1 h after meals and at bedtime	
Aluminum hydroxide	Amphojel Generic	Antacid Phosphate binder	PO: 300, 600 mg tab 320 mg/5 ml suspension	For phosphate binding: 40 ml of gel after meals and at bedtime	Constipation

RESPIRATORY DRUGS

GENERIC NAME	TRADE NAME	PREPARATIONS	GENERAL INDICATIONS	USUAL DOSAGE	CAUTIONS / COMMENTS
Bronchodilators					
Albuterol	Ventolin Proventil	PO: 2 mg tab Inhaler	Acute asthma Bronchospasm	Usual dose: 2 inhalations every 4–6 h PO: 2–4 mg 4 times daily	β_2-selective
Aminophylline		IV PO: 100, 200 mg tab Suppository: 100, 250, 500 mg	Acute asthma Bronchospasm Pulmonary edema	For acute bronchospasm IV: 5–6 mg/kg in 100 ml diluent over 20 min, followed by 1 mg/kg/h Maintenance dose: PO: 200–300 mg every 6–8 h	Reduce dosage in the elderly patients with CHF and liver disease Adverse reactions include arrhythmias, nausea, vomiting, hypotension, and seizures
Bitolterol	Tornalate	Inhaler	Acute asthma Bronchospasm	Usual dose: 2 inhalations every 8 h; more frequently for acute attack	Maximum: 2 inhalations every 4 h
Ephedrine	Generic	PO: 25, 50 mg cap	Mild asthma attack Asthma	PO: 25–50 mg every 3–4 hours	Nervousness Insomnia
Epinephrine	Medihaler-Epi	SC: 1:1000 solution Inhaler	Acute asthma Bronchospasm	SC: 0.2–0.5 ml 30 min apart up to 3 times Inhaler: 2 inhalations; may repeat in 5 min	Contraindicated in patients who are older than 50 or who have hypertension or tachycardia

Isoproterenol	Isuprel Isuprel Mistometer Medihaler-Iso	Solution: 1:100, 1:200 for nebulization Inhalers: Medihaler-Iso: 80 µg/dose Isuprel Mistometer: 131 µg/dose	Acute asthma Bronchospasm	For acute attack: Nebulizer: 0.3 ml nebulized (or diluted in 1–2 ml total volume) every 60 min up to 2 times Inhaler: 2 puffs every 3–4 h	May cause arrhythmias
Metaproterenol	Alupent Metaprel	PO: 10, 20 mg tab Inhalers	Asthma	PO: 20 mg 3–4 times daily Inhaler: 2 puffs every 4–6 h	More selective β_2 effects
Terbutaline	Brethine Bricanyl Brethaire	SC PO: 2.5, 5 mg tab Inhaler	Acute asthma Bronchospasm	SC: 0.25 mg, repeated in 15–30 min if necessary Maintenance dose: PO: 5 mg 3 times daily Inhaler: 2 inhalations every 6 h as needed	More selective β_2 effects
Theophylline	Constant-T Elixophyllin Slo-Phyllin Theo-Dur Uniphyl Others	PO: 100, 125, 200, 225, 250 mg cap; 300, 400 mg sustained-release cap IV	Asthma	PO: 200 mg 4 times daily (3–4 mg/kg every 6 h) Sustained-release: 300 mg twice daily 400 mg once daily IV: Loading dose 6 mg/kg	Effective serum concentration is 10–20 µg/ml

Table continued on following page

GENERIC NAME	TRADE NAME	PREPARATIONS	GENERAL INDICATIONS	USUAL DOSAGE	CAUTIONS/COMMENTS
Other Respiratory Agents					
Beclomethasone	Vanceril Beclovent	Inhaler	Chronic steroid-dependent asthma Allergic rhinitis	Inhaler: 2 inhalations 3–4 times daily	Of no value in treating acute attack
Cromolyn	Intal	Inhaler	Prophylactic treatment of exercise or allergen-induced asthma	Inhaler: 4 caps inhaled per day Special directions are involved	Of no value in treating acute attack
Flunisolide	AeroBid	Inhaler	Chronic steroid-dependent asthma	Inhaler: 2 inhalations twice daily	Not for acute attack
Prednisone		PO: 2.5, 5, 10, 20, 50 mg tab	Acute asthma Bronchospasm	PO: 30–60 mg daily, tapered over 3–5 days Maintenance dose: Variable	Other corticosteroids are effective
Triamcinolone	Azmacort	Inhaler	Chronic steroid-dependent asthma	Inhaler: 2 inhalations 3–4 times daily	Not for acute attack

COMBINATION DRUGS IN TREATMENT OF ASTHMA*

Combination drugs: A multitude of combination drugs are available for asthmatic patients. Generally, these drugs may be useful for patients with infrequent, easily controlled attacks.

Selected combination drugs and their ingredients are listed below. The usual dosage is one tablet or capsule 3–4 times per day.

284

Bronkotabs	Tablet: Theophylline (anhydrous) 100 mg Ephedrine 24 mg Phenobarbital 8 mg Glyceryl guaiacolate 100 mg
Marax	Tablet: Theophylline (anhydrous) 130 mg Ephedrine 25 mg Hydroxyzine (Vistaril) 10 mg Syrup (in 5 ml): 32.5, 6.25, and 2.5 mg respectively
Quadrinal	Tablet (5 ml suspension = ½ tablet): Theophylline (equivalent to 65 mg anhydrous) 130 mg Ephedrine 24 mg Phenobarbital 24 mg Potassium iodide 320 mg
Quibron	Capsule, syrup (15 ml): Theophylline (anhydrous) 150 mg Glyceryl guaiacolate 90 mg
Tedral	Tablet: Theophylline (anhydrous) 130 mg Ephedrine 24 mg Phenobarbital 8 mg
Tedral-SA	Tablet: Theophylline (anhydrous) 90 mg fast-release 90 mg slow-release Ephedrine 16 mg fast-release 32 mg slow-release Phenobarbital 25 mg (fast-release)

*From Eisenberg, M., and Copass, M.: Emergency Medical Therapy. 2nd ed. Philadelphia, W. B. Saunders Company, 1982.

RHEUMATOLOGIC DRUGS

GENERIC NAME	TRADE NAME	PREPARATIONS	GENERAL INDICATIONS	USUAL DOSAGE	CAUTIONS/COMMENTS
Antiinflammatory Drugs					
Choline salicylate	Arthropan	PO: Liquid	Rheumatoid arthritis Osteoarthritis	PO: 5 ml every 4 h	Often tolerated better than aspirin
Colchicine		IV PO: 0.5, 0.6 mg tab	Acute attack and prophylactic therapy of gout	IV: 1–2 mg initially, followed by 0.5 mg every 3–6 h PO: 0.6 mg every 1 h until symptoms subside or intolerable GI side effects occur	Avoid extravasation GI side effects are common
Diclofenac	Voltaren	PO: 25, 50, 75 mg tab	Osteoarthritis Rheumatoid arthritis	PO: 50–75 mg every 8–12 h	GI side effects
Diflunisal	Dolobid	PO: 250, 500 mg tab	Rheumatoid arthritis Osteoarthritis	PO: 500 mg every 12 h	GI side effects
Fenoprofen	Nalfon	PO: 200, 300 mg cap, 600 mg tab	Rheumatoid arthritis Osteoarthritis	PO: 200 mg every 4–6 h	GI side effects
Ibuprofen	Motrin Rufen Generic	PO: 300, 400, 600 mg tab	Rheumatoid arthritis Osteoarthritis Also approved for moderate pain	PO: 400–800 mg 4–6 times daily	GI side effects 200 mg size is available OTC

Drug	Brand	Form	Indications	Dosage	Side effects/Notes
Indomethacin	Indocin	PO: 25, 50 mg cap	Rheumatoid arthritis Ankylosing spondylitis Osteoarthritis Gout	PO: 25 mg 2–3 times daily; may increase daily dose by 25–50 mg at weekly intervals (up to 200 mg daily)	GI disturbances Ulcers Fluid retention Bone marrow depression Depression
Ketoprofen	Orudis	PO: 50, 75 mg cap	Rheumatoid arthritis Osteoarthritis	PO: 75 mg 3 times daily or 50 mg 4 times daily	GI side effects
Meclofenamate	Meclomen	PO: 50, 100 mg cap	Rheumatoid arthritis Osteoarthritis	PO: 50–100 mg 3–4 times daily	GI side effects
Naproxen	Naprosyn Anaprox	PO: 250, 375, 500 mg tab	Rheumatoid arthritis Osteoarthritis	PO: 250 mg 3 times daily	GI side effects
Oxyphenbutazone	Oxalid Tandearil	PO: 100 mg tab	Acute attack of gout Also useful for: Rheumatoid arthritis Osteoarthritis Ankylosing spondylitis	PO: 200 mg every 6 h, then taper over 3–5 days	GI disturbances Rash Fluid retention Bone marrow depression Chronic use should be undertaken with caution
Phenylbutazone	Azolid Butazolidin	PO: 100 mg tab			
Piroxicam	Feldene	PO: 10, 20 mg cap	Rheumatoid arthritis Osteoarthritis	PO: 10–20 mg daily	GI side effects
Salicylate (Aspirin)	Many names	PO: 65, 162, 325, 650 mg tab	Rheumatoid arthritis Osteoarthritis	Must be individualized	Drug of choice for rheumatoid arthritis and osteoarthritis
Sulindac	Clinoril	PO: 150, 200 mg tab	Inflammatory arthritis	PO: 150 mg twice daily	GI disturbances
Suprofen	Suprol	PO: 200 mg cap	Osteoarthritis, second line drug	PO: 200 mg every 4–6 h	Renal toxicity

Table continued on following page

GENERIC NAME	TRADE NAME	PREPARATIONS	GENERAL INDICATIONS	USUAL DOSAGE	CAUTIONS/COMMENTS
Tolmetin	Tolectin	PO: 200 mg tab, 400 mg cap	Rheumatoid arthritis	PO: 400 mg 3 times daily initially Maintenance dose: 600 mg–1.8 g daily	GI disturbances
Uric Acid–Lowering Drugs					
Allopurinol	Zyloprim	PO: 100, 300 mg tab	Chronic gout Secondary hyperuricemia	For gout: PO: 200–400 mg in single daily dose For secondary hyperuricemia: PO: 100–300 mg daily	Not for treatment of acute attacks Use colchicine for several days when initiating therapy
Probenecid	Benemid	PO: 500 mg tab	Chronic gout	PO: 500 mg 2–3 times daily initially, then adjust for maintenance	GI disturbances Not for treatment of acute attacks Avoid in patients with renal failure or kidney stones
Sulfinpyrazone	Anturane	PO: 100 mg tab	Chronic gout	PO: 100–200 mg twice daily given with food; gradually increase up to 800 mg daily to control serious uric acid level	ASA diminishes the activity of sulfinpyrazone; the drugs should not be used concurrently Use colchicine for several days when initiating therapy

INDEX

Note: Page numbers followed by t refer to tabulated material.

298 / INDEX